QUICK GUIDE
TO SOLVING PROBLEMS
Using Dimensional Analysis

QUICK GUIDE
TO SOLVING PROBLEMS
Using Dimensional Analysis

Gloria P. Craig, RN, MSN, EdD
Department Head, Nursing Student Services
Assistant Professor, College of Nursing
South Dakota State University
Brookings, South Dakota

DISCARD

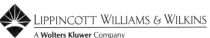

LIPPINCOTT WILLIAMS & WILKINS
A **Wolters Kluwer** Company
Philadelphia · Baltimore · New York · London
Buenos Aires · Hong Kong · Sydney · Tokyo

Acquisitions Editor: Margaret Zuccarini
Senior Editorial Coordinator: Helen Kogut
Senior Production Editor: Debra Schiff
Senior Production Manager: Helen Ewan
Managing Editor / Production: Erika Kors
Design Coordinator: Marie Clifton
Manufacturing Manager: William Alberti
Indexer: Angie Wiley
Compositor: Circle Graphics
Printer: R.R. Donnelley

9 8 7 6 5 4 3 2 1

Library of Congress Cataloging-in-Publication Data

Craig, Gloria P., 1949-
  Quick guide to solving problems using dimensional analysis / Gloria P. Craig.
    p. cm.
  Includes index.
  ISBN 0-7817-4018-5 (alk. paper)
    1. Pharmaceutical arithmetic. 2. Dimensional analysis. I. Title.

RS57 .C733 2003
615′.1′0151—dc21

2002016149

LWW.com

Kari R. Lane, RN, BSN, MSN
Nursing Instructor
Clinton Community College
Eastern Iowa Community College District
Clinton, Iowa

Francine P. Pappalardo, BSN, MSN
Professor
Northern Essex Community College
Lawrence, Massachusetts

Terri M. Perkins, RN, MN
Instructor, Associate Degree Nursing Program
Bellevue Community College
Bellevue, Washington

Peggy Anne Przybycien, RN, BSN, MSN, CNS
Assistant Professor
Onondaga Community College
Syracuse, New York

Alice Rasmussen, RN, MSN
Nursing Coordinator and Health Science
    Department Chair
Lake Michigan College
Benton Harbor, Michigan

Laura Sessions, RN, MScN
Instructor of Nursing
Howard Community College
Columbia, Maryland

Jo A. Voss, RN, BSN, MSN
Nursing Instructor
South Dakota State University
Rapid City, South Dakota

Medication errors continue to be a significant problem in our health care system. The error rate can be reduced through use of a problem-solving method that is easy to understand. Many people have difficulty calculating mathematical problems due to mathematical deficiencies sometimes leading to "math anxiety." Most medication errors are made because the medication problems are set up incorrectly, resulting in an inaccurate dosage of medication administered to the patient.

As a student nurse, I had difficulty with medication calculations because of high anxiety related to mathematical deficiencies. A friend introduced me to a problem-solving method that was easy for me to understand and allowed me to visualize all parts of the medication problem. This one problem-solving method allowed me to solve a variety of medication problems. Instead of memorizing a formula, I was able to focus on seeing and understanding all of the components necessary in the medication problems. This problem-solving method was what we now know as dimensional analysis.

As a student nurse, I created a "little book" to carry in my pocket that contained examples of medication problems that might be encountered in the clinical setting. Each new medication problem that I encountered was judiciously added to my "little book" for future reference. As a visual learner, this "little book" enriched my clinical experience by providing numerous illustrations of medication problems. Soon, other students were asking to use my "little book."

Dimensional analysis is a problem-solving method that can eliminate the stumbling blocks related to a lack of mathematical abilities or anxiety and empower the learner to solve a variety of medication calculation problems utilizing one problem-solving method. This pocket reference begins in **Chapter 1** by assisting the learner with an arithmetic review of the mathematical skills that will be necessary to calculate medication problems using dimensional analysis. Following the arithmetic review, **Chapter 2** provides the learner with information regarding the different systems of measurement and common equivalents used in medication administration. **Chapter 3** introduces the learner to dimensional analysis as a problem-solving method and **Chapter 4** provides various types of realistic medication problems before advancing the learner to the more complex medication problems in **Chapters 5** and **6**. **Chapter 7** reinforces the learner by providing ample practice answering a variety of medication calculation problems to build confidence and ability. The text also provides not only answers to the medication problems, but demonstrates "how" the answers were obtained by illustrating "how" to set up of the medication problem.

This pocket-sized text can be easily carried in the pocket of a uniform jacket as a quick reference for students. The front inside cover contains terms used with dimensional analysis, the five steps necessary to solve a problem using dimensional analysis, and an illustration of the Unit Path used in solving problems with dimensional analysis. The back inside cover contains volume and weight equivalents information.

As a method of reducing medication errors and improving medication dosage calculation abilities, dimensional analysis offers much promise. As we learn more about learning styles and disabilities, problem solving with dimensional analysis becomes more meaningful as it empowers the learner to understand "how to learn" rather than "what to learn" and supports higher-level thinking skills that are necessary to be a safe, effective nurse in the 21st century.

Recently, while going through my library, I ran across that tattered and torn "little book" and remembered what a valuable learning tool it had been for me during my years as a student nurse. It is my dream to share this "little book" with others who need a visual reference for a consistent problem-solving method that can be used to set up a variety of medication calculation problems.

Gloria P. Craig

Acknowledgments

There are many people who have assisted me with my professional growth and development including:

- **Pauline Callahan**, who believed that I would be a great nurse and nursing instructor when I could not believe in myself.

- **Jackie Kehm**, who introduced me to dimensional analysis and helped me pass the medication module that I was sure would be my stumbling block.

- **Dr. Sandra L. Sellers**, for her expertise and guidance throughout the process of writing my thesis and her encouragement to write a textbook.

- **Margaret Cooper**, for her friendship and editing support throughout the writing of *Clinical Calculations Made Easy*, 2e.

- My students, colleagues, and reviewers for helping me develop my abilities to explain and teach the problem-solving method of dimensional analysis.

- The numerous pharmaceutical companies listed throughout this book that supplied medication labels and gave permission for the labels to be included in this textbook.

- The faculty at South Dakota State University, College of Nursing for allowing dimensional analysis to be integrated into the curriculum as the problem-solving method for medication calculation.

- The Lippincott editorial and production teams, for all of their hard work: **Margaret Zuccarini,** Senior Acquisitions Editor; **Helen Kogut,** Senior Editorial

Coordinator; **Debra Schiff,** Senior Production Editor; and **Marie Clifton,** Design Coordinator.

To these people and many more, I would like to express my sincere appreciation for their mentoring, guidance, support, and encouragement that have helped to turn a dream into a reality.

Contents

ARITHMETIC REVIEW

This chapter provides a review of the basic mathematical concepts that you will need to calculate dosages using dimensional analysis. This chapter will review Arabic numbers, Roman numerals, fractions, and decimals. You will have an opportunity to practice multiplication and division of fractions and decimals as well as conversion of fractions to decimals.

ARABIC NUMBERS AND ROMAN NUMERALS

- The physician or nurse practitioner orders most medication dosages in the metric and household systems for weights and measures using the Arabic number system with symbols called **digits** (1, 2, 3, 4, 5).
- Orders are also received in the apothecary system of weights and measures using the Roman numeral system with numbers represented by **symbols** (I, V, X). The Roman numeral system uses seven basic symbols with a combination of symbols representing all numbers in the Arabic number system.

Table 1.1 includes the seven basic **Roman numerals** and the corresponding **Arabic numbers.**

The combination of Roman numerals symbols is based upon three specific principles.

- The **first principle** is that symbols are used to construct a number but no symbol may be used more than three times. The exception is the symbol for five (V) that is used only once because there is a symbol for 10 (X) and a combination of symbols for 15 (XV).

EXAMPLE 1.1

III = (1 + 1 + 1) = 3

XXX = (10 + 10 + 10) = 30

● Table 1.1 Basic Roman Numerals and Arabic Numbers

ROMAN NUMERALS	ARABIC NUMBERS
I	1
V	5
X	10
L	50
C	100
D	500
M	1000

- The **second principle** is that symbols of lesser value following symbols of greater value are **added** to construct a number.

EXAMPLE 1.2

VIII = (5 + 3) = 8
XVII = (10 + 5 + 1 + 1) = 17

- The **third principle** is that symbols of greater value following symbols of lesser value are **subtracted** to construct a number.

EXAMPLE 1.3

IV = (1 − 5) = 4
IX = (1 − 10) = 9

Practice Exercise 1.1   Roman Numerals to Arabic Numbers

Express the following Roman numerals as Arabic numbers.

1. II   = _____
2. IV   = _____
3. VI   = _____
4. X   = _____
5. VIII = _____

6. XIX = _____
7. XX = _____
8. XVIII = _____
9. I = _____
10. XV = _____
11. III = _____
12. V = _____
13. IX = _____
14. VII = _____
15. XI = _____
16. XIV = _____
17. XVI = _____
18. XII = _____
19. XVII = _____
20. XIII = _____

Practice Exercise 1.2 Converting Arabic Numbers and Roman Numerals

To increase your ability to utilize either system, convert the following Arabic numbers or Roman numerals.

1. 34 = _____
2. XXII = _____
3. 75 = _____
4. XC = _____
5. 29 = _____
6. XLII = _____
7. 56 = _____
8. LXIV = _____
9. 88 = _____
10. CXXI = _____

FRACTIONS

Medication dosages with fractions are occasionally ordered by the physician or nurse practitioner or used by pharmaceutical manufacturers on the drug label. A

fraction is a number that represents part of a whole number and contains three parts:

- **Numerator**—the number on the top portion of the fraction and represents the number of parts of the whole fraction.
- **Dividing line**—the line separating the top portion of the fraction from the bottom portion of the fraction.
- **Denominator**—the number on the bottom portion of the fraction and represents the number of parts into which the whole is divided.

EXAMPLE 1.4

$\dfrac{3}{4} = \dfrac{\text{numerator}}{\text{denominator}}$

To solve medication dosage calculation problems using dimensional analysis, you must be able to identify the numerator and denominator portion of the problem. You also must be able to multiply and divide numbers, fractions, and decimals.

Multiplying Fractions

There are three steps involved in multiplying fractions.

- **Step One:** Multiply the numerators.
- **Step Two:** Multiply the denominators.
- **Step Three:** Reduce the product to the lowest possible fraction.

EXAMPLE 1.5

$$\frac{1}{2} \times \frac{2}{4} = \frac{2}{8} = \frac{1}{4}$$

$$\frac{1 \times 2 = 2 \,(\text{divided by } 2) = 1}{2 \times 4 = 8 \,(\text{divided by } 2) = 4} \text{ or } \frac{1}{4}$$

$$\frac{1 \,(\text{numerator}) \ \times 2 \,(\text{numerator}) \ = 2 \,(\text{numerator}) \ = 1}{2 \,(\text{denominator}) \times 4 \,(\text{denominator}) = 8 \,(\text{denominator}) = 4}$$

or $\dfrac{1}{4}$

Practice Exercise 1.3 Multiplying Fractions

To increase your ability to work with fractions, multiply the following fractions and reduce to the lowest fractional terms.

1. $\dfrac{3}{4} \times \dfrac{5}{8} =$

2. $\dfrac{1}{3} \times \dfrac{4}{9} =$

3. $\dfrac{2}{3} \times \dfrac{4}{5} =$

4. $\dfrac{3}{4} \times \dfrac{1}{2} =$

5. $\dfrac{1}{8} \times \dfrac{4}{5} =$

6. $\dfrac{2}{3} \times \dfrac{5}{8} =$

7. $\dfrac{3}{8} \times \dfrac{2}{3} =$

8. $\dfrac{4}{7} \times \dfrac{2}{4} =$

9. $\dfrac{4}{5} \times \dfrac{1}{2} =$

10. $\dfrac{1}{4} \times \dfrac{1}{8} =$

Dividing Fractions

There are four steps involved in dividing fractions.

- **Step 1:** Invert (turn upside down) the divisor portion of the problem (the second fraction in the problem).
- **Step 2:** Multiply the two numerators.
- **Step 3:** Multiply the two denominators.
- **Step 4:** Reduce the answer to the lowest term (fraction or whole number).

EXAMPLE 1.6

$$\frac{1}{2} \div \frac{2}{4} = \frac{1}{2} \times \frac{4}{2} = \frac{4}{4} = 1$$

$$\frac{1\,(\text{numerator})}{2\,(\text{denominator})} \div \frac{2\,(\text{numerator})}{4\,(\text{denominator})}$$

$$= \frac{1\,(\text{numerator}) \quad \times \quad \overset{(\textit{inverted fraction})}{4}\,(\text{numerator}) \;=\; 4}{2\,(\text{denominator}) \;\times\; 2\,(\text{denominator}) \;=\; 4}$$

$$= 1\,(\text{answer reduced to lowest term})$$

Practice Exercise 1.4   Dividing Fractions

To increase your ability to work with fractions, divide the following fractions and reduce to the lowest fractional terms.

1. $\dfrac{3}{4} \div \dfrac{2}{3} =$

2. $\dfrac{1}{9} \div \dfrac{3}{9} =$

3. $\dfrac{2}{3} \div \dfrac{1}{6} =$

4. $\dfrac{1}{5} \div \dfrac{4}{5} =$

5. $\dfrac{3}{6} \div \dfrac{4}{8} =$

6. $\dfrac{5}{8} \div \dfrac{5}{8} =$

7. $\dfrac{1}{8} \div \dfrac{2}{3} =$

8. $\dfrac{1}{5} \div \dfrac{1}{2} =$

DECIMALS

Medication orders are often written using decimals, and pharmaceutical manufacturers may use decimals when labeling medications. Therefore, you must understand the specific principles involving decimals and be able to multiply and divide decimals.

- A decimal point is preceded by a zero if not preceded by a number to decrease chance of an error if the decimal point is missed.

EXAMPLE 1.7
0.25

- A decimal point may be preceded by a number and followed by a number.

EXAMPLE 1.8
1.25

- Numbers to the left of the decimal point are *units, tens, hundreds, thousands,* and *ten-thousands.*
- Numbers to the right of the decimal point are *tenths, hundredths, thousandths,* and *ten-thousandths.*

EXAMPLE 1.9

0.2 = 2 tenths

0.05 = 5 hundredths

0.25 = 25 hundredths

1.25 = 1 unit and 25 hundredths

110.25 = one hundred ten and 25 hundredths

Rounding Decimals

- Decimals may be rounded off. If the number to the right of the decimal is greater than or equal to 5 (≥ 5), round up to the next number.
- If the number to the right of the decimal is less than 5 (≤ 5), delete the remaining numbers.

EXAMPLE 1.10

0.213 = 0.2

Practice Exercise 1.5   Rounding Decimals

Practice rounding off the following decimals to the tenth.

1. 0.75 =
2. 0.88 =
3. 0.44 =
4. 0.23 =
5. 0.67 =
6. 0.27 =
7. 0.98 =
8. 0.92 =

Multiplying Decimals

When multiplying with decimals, the principles of multiplication will still apply. The numbers are multiplied in columns but the number of decimal points are counted and placed in the answer counting places from right to left.

EXAMPLE 1.11

```
  2.3   (1 decimal point)
× 1.5   (1 decimal point)
  115
  230
  3.45  (2 decimal points added to the answer,
         counting 2 places from the right to left)
```

Practice Exercise 1.6 Multiplying Decimals

Practice multiplying the following decimals.

1.   2.5
    × 4.6

2.   1.45
    × 0.25

3.   3.9
    × 0.8

4.   2.56
    × 0.45

5.   10.65
    × 0.05

6.   1.98
    × 3.10

Dividing Decimals

When dividing with decimals, the principles of division still apply except that the dividing number is changed to a whole number by moving the decimal point to the right. The number being divided also changes by accepting the same number of decimal point moves.

EXAMPLE 1.12

$0.5\overline{)0.75}$

- Step 1: Move the decimal point one place to the right for both of the numbers.

- Step 2:
$$
\begin{array}{r}
1.5 \\
05\overline{)7.5} \\
\underline{5} \\
2.5 \\
\underline{2\,5} \\
0
\end{array}
$$

Practice Exercise 1.7   Dividing Decimals

Practice dividing the following decimals and rounding the answer to the tenth.

1. $3.4\overline{)9.6}$

2. $0.25\overline{)12.50}$

3. $0.56\overline{)18.65}$

4. $0.3\overline{)0.192}$

5. $0.4\overline{)12.43}$

6. $0.5\overline{)12.50}$

7. $0.125\overline{)0.25}$

8. $0.08\overline{)0.085}$

CONVERTING FRACTIONS TO DECIMALS

When solving problems using dimensional analysis, medication problems may frequently contain both fractions and decimals. Some of you may have **fraction phobia** and prefer to convert fractions to decimals when solving problems. To convert a fraction to a decimal, divide the numerator portion of the fraction by the denominator portion of the fraction. When dividing fractions, remember to add a decimal point and a zero if the numerator cannot be divided by the denominator.

EXAMPLE 1.13

$$\frac{1}{2} \text{ or } \frac{1 \,(\text{numerator})}{2 \,(\text{denominator})} = 2\overline{)1.0} = 0.5 \quad \begin{array}{c} 0.5 \\ \underline{1\,0} \end{array}$$

Practice Exercise 1.8 Converting Fractions to Decimals

To decrease fraction phobia, practice converting the following fractions to decimals.

1. $\dfrac{1}{8}$ =

2. $\dfrac{1}{4}$ =

3. $\dfrac{2}{5}$ =

(continued)

Practice Exercise 1.8 Converting Fractions in Decimals
(Continued)

4. $\dfrac{3}{5}$ =

5. $\dfrac{2}{3}$ =

6. $\dfrac{6}{8}$ =

7. $\dfrac{3}{8}$ =

8. $\dfrac{1}{3}$ =

9. $\dfrac{3}{6}$ =

10. $\dfrac{2}{10}$ =

SUMMARY

Chapter 1 has reviewed **basic mathematics** that will assist you to successfully implement dimensional analysis as a problem-solving method for medication dosage calculations.

SYSTEMS OF MEASUREMENT AND COMMON EQUIVALENTS

This chapter will help you to understand the measurement systems used for medication administration. You will need to understand common equivalents and units of measurement to visualize all parts of a medication dosage calculation problem. This knowledge is necessary to accurately implement the problem-solving method of dimensional analysis.

SYSTEMS OF MEASUREMENT

There are three systems of measurement used for medication dosage administration:

- The **metric system**
- The **apothecary system**
- The **household system.**

To be able to accurately administer medication, it is necessary to understand all three of these systems.

Metric System

The **metric system** is a decimal system of weights and measures based on units of ten in which gram, meter, and liter are the basic units of measurement.

- Gram and liter are the measurements from the metric system that are most frequently used in medication administration.
- Meter is a unit of distance and is not typically used in medication administration.
- Gram (abbreviated g or gm) is a unit of weight.
- Liter (abbreviated L) is a unit of volume.

Frequently used metric weight units are summarized in **Box 2.1.**

Box 2.1   **Metric System Units of Weight and Equivalents**

1 kilogram (kg)
1 gram (g)
1 milligram (mg)
1 microgram (mcg)
1 kg = 1000 g
1 g = 1000 mg
1 mg = 1000 mcg

The most frequently used volume measurements and equivalents within the metric system are summarized in **Box 2.2** and displayed in **Figure 2.1**.

Box 2.2   **Metric System Units of Volume and Equivalents**

1 liter (L)
1 milliliter (mL)
1 cubic centimeter (cc)
1 L = 1000 mL
1 mL = 1 cc

Practice Exercise 2.1   Metric System

Write the correct abbreviation symbols for the following measurements from the metric system:

1. kilogram   =
2. gram   =
3. milligram   =
4. microgram   =
5. liter   =
6. milliliter   =
7. cubic centimeter =

Weight: Basic unit is gram (g)

Equivalents:
- Kilogram (kg)   1 kg = 1,000 g
- Milligram (mg   1 mg = 1/1,000 g
- Microgram (mcg)   1mcg = 1/1,000 mg = 1/1,000,000 g

Volume: Basic unit is liter (L)

Equivalents:
- Milliliter (mL)   1 mL = 1/1,000 L
- Cubic centimeter (cc)   1 cc = 1 mL = 1/1,000 L

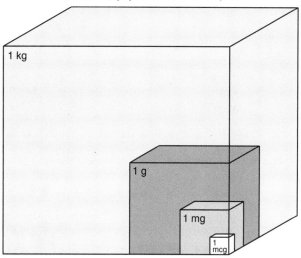

Figure 2.1 Metric units frequently used for drug administration. Another way to understand metric equivalents is to visualize the relationships between equivalent measurements. Please note that the figure is not drawn to scale.

Apothecary System

The **apothecary system** is a system of measuring and weighing drugs and solutions in which fractions are used to identify parts of the unit of measure. The basic units of measurement in the apothecary system include:

- Weights
- Liquid volume

Although the apothecary system may be replaced by the metric system, it is still necessary to understand this system because some physicians continue to order medications using this system and also may include Roman numerals in the medication order.

The most frequently used weight measurements and equivalents within the apothecary system are summarized in **Box 2.3** and displayed in **Figure 2.2.**

Box 2.3 **Apothecary System Units of Weight and Equivalents**

1 pound (lb)
1 ounce (oz)
1 dram (dr)
1 grain (gr)
1 lb = 16 oz
1 oz = 8 dr
1 dr = 60 gr

The most frequently used volume measurements and equivalents within the apothecary system are summarized in **Box 2.4** and displayed in **Figure 2.2.**

Box 2.4 **Apothecary System Units of Volume and Equivalents**

1 gallon (gal)
1 quart (qt)
1 pint (pt)
1 fluid ounce (fl oz)
1 fluid dram (fl dr)
1 minim (M)
1 gal = 4 qt
1 qt = 2 pt
1 pt = 16 fl oz
1 fl oz = 8 fl dr
1 fl dr = 60 M
1 fl oz = 1 oz
1 fl dr = 1 dr

Weight

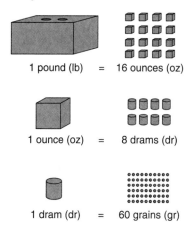

1 pound (lb)   =   16 ounces (oz)

1 ounce (oz)   =   8 drams (dr)

1 dram (dr)   =   60 grains (gr)

Volume

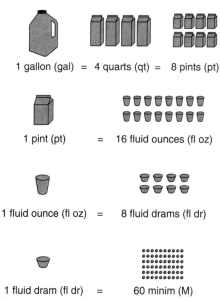

1 gallon (gal)   =   4 quarts (qt)   =   8 pints (pt)

1 pint (pt)   =   16 fluid ounces (fl oz)

1 fluid ounce (fl oz)   =   8 fluid drams (fl dr)

1 fluid dram (fl dr)   =   60 minim (M)

Figure 2.2 Apothecary system of equivalents for weight and volume. Please note that the figures are not shown to scale.

Practice Exercise 2.2 Apothecary System

Write the correct abbreviation symbols for the following measurements from the apothecary system:

1. pound   =
2. ounce   =
3. dram   =
4. grain   =
5. gallon   =
6. quart   =
7. pint   =
8. fluid ounce =
9. fluid dram =
10. minim   =

Household Measurements

The use of **household measurements** is considered inaccurate because of the varying sizes of cups, glasses, and eating utensils, and this system has generally been replaced with the metric system. However, with patient care moving away from hospitals using the metric system and into the community, it is once again necessary for the nurse to have an understanding of the household measurement system to be able to utilize and teach this system to clients and families.

The most frequently used measurements and equivalents within the household measurement system are summarized in **Box 2.5** and displayed in **Figure 2.3**.

> ## Box 2.5 Household Measurement System and Equivalents
>
> 1 glass
> 1 cup
> 1 tablespoon (tbsp or T)
> 1 teaspoon (tsp or t)
> 1 drop (gtt)
> 1 glass or cup = 8 ounces (oz)
> 1 teacup = 6 ounces (oz)
> 2 tbsp = 1 oz
> 3 tsp = 1 tbsp
> 1 tsp = 60 gtt

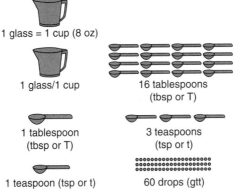

1 glass = 1 cup (8 oz)

1 glass/1 cup

16 tablespoons (tbsp or T)

1 tablespoon (tbsp or T)

3 teaspoons (tsp or t)

1 teaspoon (tsp or t)

60 drops (gtt)

Figure 2.3 Household measurement system and equivalents for volume. Please note that the figures are not shown to scale.

Practice Exercise 2.3   Household System

Write the correct abbreviation symbols for the following measurements from the household system:

1. tablespoon   =
2. teaspoon   =
3. drop   =

System Equivalents

Sometimes it is necessary to convert from one system to another to be able to accurately administer medication. **Table 2.1** summarizes the most frequently used measurements and lists the approximate equivalents in the metric, apothecary, and household systems.

● Table 2.1 Approximate Equivalents		
METRIC	APOTHECARY	HOUSEHOLD
4000 mL	1 gal (4 qt)	
1 L (1000 mL)	1 qt (2 pt)	
500 mL	1 pt (16 fl oz)	
240 mL	8 oz	1 glass/coffee cup
180 mL	6 oz	1 cup (teacup)
30 mL	1 oz (8 dr)	2 tbsp
15 mL	½ oz (4 dr)	1 tbsp (3 tsp)
5 mL	1 dr (60 M)	1 tsp (60 gtt)
1 mL (1 cc)	15 M	15 gtt
	1 M	1 gtt

Practice Exercise 2.4 Equivalents

Identify the correct numerical values for the following measurements:

1. 1 kg = _____ lb
2. 1 kg = _____ g
3. 1 g = _____ mg
4. 1 mg = _____ mcg
5. 1 g = _____ gr
6. 1 gr = _____ mg
7. 1000 mg = _____ g
8. 1000 mL = _____ L = _____ qt
9. 500 mL = _____ pt
10. 240 mL = _____ oz
11. 30 mL = _____ oz = _____ tbsp
12. 15 mL = _____ oz = _____ tsp
13. 5 mL = _____ tsp
14. 1 mL = _____ M = _____ gtt
15. 1 mL = _____ cc

SUMMARY

Chapter 2 has helped you review the **measurement systems** used for medication administration including the **metric system,** the **apothecary system,** and the **household system.**

SOLVING PROBLEMS USING DIMENSIONAL ANALYSIS

3

This chapter introduces you to dimensional analysis with a step-by-step explanation of this problem-solving method. Dimensional analysis provides a systematic straightforward way to set up problems. It is not only easy to learn, but also can reduce errors when mathematical conversion is required. This system allows conceptualization of a problem through visualization of all its parts using critical thinking. This chapter also provides the opportunity to practice solving problems involving common equivalents.

TERMS USED WITH DIMENSIONAL ANALYSIS

Dimensional analysis is a problem-solving method that can be used whenever two quantities are directly proportional to each other and one quantity must be converted to the other using a common equivalent, conversion factor, or conversion relation. All medication dosage calculation problems can be solved with dimensional analysis.

It is important to understand the following four terms that provide the basis for dimensional analysis.

- **Given quantity:** the beginning point of the problem.
- **Wanted quantity:** the answer to the problem.
- **Unit path:** the series of conversions necessary to achieve the answer to the problem.
- **Conversion factors:** equivalents necessary to convert between systems of measurement and allow unwanted units to be canceled from the problem. Each conversion factor is a ratio of units that equals 1.

Dimensional analysis also uses the same terms as fractions: **numerators** and **denominators.**
- *The numerator* = the top portion of the problem.
- *The denominator* = the bottom portion of the problem.

Some problems will have a given quantity and a wanted quantity that contain only numerators. Other problems will have a given quantity and a wanted quantity that contain both a numerator and a denominator. This chapter contains only problems with numerators as the given quantity and the wanted quantity.

Once the beginning point in the problem is identified, then a series of conversions necessary to achieve the answer is established, leading to the problem's solution. Below is an example of the problem-solving method, showing the placement of basic terms used in dimensional analysis.

	Unit Path			
Given Quantity	Conversion Factor for Given Quantity	Conversion Factor for Wanted Quantity	Conversion Computation	Wanted Quantity
1 liter (L)	1000 mL	1 oz	$1 \times 1000 \times 1$	1000
	1 liter (L)	30 mL	1×30	$\dfrac{1000}{30} = 33.3$ oz

THE FIVE STEPS OF DIMENSIONAL ANALYSIS

Once the given quantity is identified, the unit path leading to the wanted quantity is established. The problem-solving method of dimensional analysis can be explained using the following five steps.

- **Step 1:** Identify the *given quantity* in the problem.
- **Step 2:** Identify the *wanted quantity* in the problem.
- **Step 3:** Establish the *unit path* from the given quantity to the wanted quantity using equivalents as *conversion factors*.
- **Step 4:** Set up the problem to allow for cancellation of unwanted units. Carefully choose each conversion factor and ensure that it is correctly placed in the numerator or denominator portion of the problem to

allow the unwanted units to be canceled from the problem.
• **Step 5:** Multiply the numerators, multiply the denominators, and divide the product of the numerators by the product of the denominators to provide the numerical value of the wanted quantity.

The following examples use the five steps to solve a problem using dimensional analysis.

EXAMPLE 3.1

1 liter equals how many ounces. Or: How many ounces are in 1 liter?

Step 1: Identify the *given quantity* in the problem.
Need to Know: What is the given quantity?
Answer: The given quantity is *1 liter* (L).

$$\frac{1 \text{ liter}}{} =$$

Step 2: Identify the *wanted quantity* in the problem.
Need to Know: What is the wanted quantity?
Answer: The wanted quantity is the number of *ounces* (oz) in 1 liter.

$$\frac{1 \text{ liter}}{} = \quad \text{ounces}$$

Step 3: Establish the *unit path* from the given quantity to the wanted quantity by selecting the equivalents that will be used as conversion factors.
Need to Know: What conversion factors are needed in the unit path that will convert the given quantity to the wanted quantity?
Answer:
given quantity of 1 liter (L) = 1000 mL
wanted quantity of 1 ounce (oz) = 30 mL

$$\frac{1 \text{ liter (L)}}{} = \quad \text{ounces (oz)}$$

Step 4: Write the unit path for the problem so that each unit cancels out the preceding unit until all unwanted units are canceled from the problem except the wanted quantity.

Need to Know: What is the wanted quantity that remains in the unit path after canceling all unwanted units?

Answer:

1 liter (L)	1000 mL	1 (oz)	
	1 liter (L)	30 mL	= ounces

Step 5: After the unwanted units are canceled from the problem, only the numerical values remain. Multiply the numerators, multiply the denominators, and divide the product of the numerators by the product of the denominators to provide the numerical value for the wanted quantity. One (1) times ($\times$) any number equals that number, therefore ones (1s) may be automatically canceled from the problem. Other factors that can be canceled from the problem include like numerical values in the numerator and denominator portion of the problem and the same number of zeroes (0s) in the numerator and denominator portion of the problem.

Need to Know:

What is the product of the numerators?

What is the product of the denominators?

After multiplying the numerators and the denominators, and dividing the product of the numerators by the product of the denominators, what is the numerical value for the wanted quantity?

Answer:

1 L	1000 mL	1 (oz)	1 × 1000 × 1	1000	
	1 L	30 mL	1 × 30	30	= 33.3 ounces

33.3 ounces is the wanted quantity and the answer to the problem. Another example of the problem-solving method of dimensional analysis is summarized as follows:

EXAMPLE 3.2

One gallon equals how many milliliters? Or: How many milliliters are in one gallon?

Step 1: Identify the given quantity in the problem.

Need to Know: What is the given quantity?

Answer: The given quantity is *one gallon*.

$$\frac{1 \text{ gallon}}{} \qquad = $$

Step 2: Identify the wanted quantity in the problem.

Need to Know: What is the wanted quantity?

Answer: The wanted quantity is the number of *milliliters* in one gallon.

$$\frac{1 \text{ gallon}}{} \qquad = \qquad \text{milliliters}$$

Step 3: Establish the unit path from the given quantity to the wanted quantity by selecting the equivalents that will be used as conversion factors.

Need to Know: What conversion factors are needed in the unit path that will convert the given quantity to the wanted quantity?

Answer:

Given quantity of 1 gallon = 4 quarts

4 quarts = 1 liter

1 liter = 1000 mL (the wanted quantity unit)

Step 4: Write the unit path for the problem so that each unit cancels out the preceding unit until all unwanted units are canceled from the problem except the wanted quantity.

Need to Know: What is the wanted quantity that remains in the unit path after canceling all unwanted units?

$$\frac{1 \;\cancel{\text{gal}}}{} \; \left| \; \frac{4 \;\cancel{\text{qt}}}{1 \;\cancel{\text{gal}}} \; \right| \; \frac{1 \;\cancel{\text{L}}}{1 \;\cancel{\text{qt}}} \; \left| \; \frac{1000 \;(\text{mL})}{1 \;\cancel{\text{L}}} \right| \; = \; \text{mL}$$

Step 5: After the unwanted units are canceled from the problem, only the numerical values remain. Multiply the numerators, multiply the denominators, and divide the product of the numerators by the product of the denominators to provide the numerical value for the wanted quantity.

Need to Know: What is the product of the numerators? What is the product of the denominators?

After multiplying the numerators and the denominators, and dividing the product of the numerators by the product of the denominators, what is the numerical value for the wanted quantity?

Answer:

~~4 gal~~	4 qt	4 ~~L~~	1000 (mL)	4 × 1000	= 4000 mL
	~~4 gal~~	1 qt	4 ~~L~~	1	

Practice Exercise 3.1 Using Dimensional Analysis

Use dimensional analysis to change the following units of measurement.

1. Problem: 4 mg   =   How many g?
   Given quantity   =
   Wanted quantity   =

$$\frac{4\text{ mg}}{\vert} = \qquad \text{g}$$

2. Problem: 5000 g   =   How many kg?
   Given quantity   =
   Wanted quantity   =

$$\frac{5000\text{ g}}{\vert} = \qquad \text{kg}$$

3. Problem: 0.3 L   =   How many cc?
   Given quantity   =
   Wanted quantity   =

$$\frac{0.3\text{ L}}{\vert} = \qquad \text{cc}$$

4. Problem: 10 cc   =   How many mL?
   Given quantity   =
   Wanted quantity   =

$$\frac{10\text{ cc}}{\vert} = \qquad \text{mL}$$

5. Problem: 120 lb   =   How many kg?
   Given quantity   =
   Wanted quantity   =

$$\frac{120\ lb\ |}{|\rule{7cm}{0pt}} = \quad kg$$

6. Problem: 5 gr   =   How many mg?
   Given quantity   =
   Wanted quantity =

$$\frac{5\ gr\ |}{|\rule{7cm}{0pt}} = \quad mg$$

7. Problem: 2 g   =   How many gr?
   Given quantity =
   Wanted quantity =

$$\frac{2\ g\ |}{|\rule{7cm}{0pt}} = \quad gr$$

8. Problem: 5 fl dr   =   How many mL?
   Given quantity   =
   Wanted quantity   =

$$\frac{5\ fl\ dr\ |}{|\rule{7cm}{0pt}} = \quad mL$$

9. Problem: 8 fl dr   =   How many fl oz?
   Given quantity   =
   Wanted quantity   =

$$\frac{8\ fl\ dr\ |}{|\rule{7cm}{0pt}} = \quad fl\ oz$$

10. Problem: 10 M   =   How many fl dr?
    Given quantity   =
    Wanted quantity =

$$\frac{10\ M\ |}{|\rule{7cm}{0pt}} = \quad fl\ dr$$

(continued)

Practice Exercise 3.1 Using Dimensional Analysis
(Continued)

11. Problem: 35 kg = How many lb?
    Given quantity =
    Wanted quantity =

$$\frac{35 \text{ kg}}{\rule{5cm}{0pt}} = \rule{2cm}{0pt} \text{lb}$$

12. Problem: 10 mL = How many tsp?
    Given quantity =
    Wanted quantity =

$$\frac{10 \text{ mL}}{\rule{5cm}{0pt}} = \rule{2cm}{0pt} \text{tsp}$$

13. Problem: 30 mL = How many tbsp?
    Given quantity =
    Wanted quantity =

$$\frac{30 \text{ mL}}{\rule{5cm}{0pt}} = \rule{2cm}{0pt} \text{tbsp}$$

14. Problem: 0.25 g = How many mg?
    Given quantity =
    Wanted quantity =

$$\frac{0.25 \text{ g}}{\rule{5cm}{0pt}} = \rule{2cm}{0pt} \text{mg}$$

15. Problem: 350 mcg = How many mg?
    Given quantity =
    Wanted quantity =

$$\frac{350 \text{ mcg}}{\rule{5cm}{0pt}} = \rule{2cm}{0pt} \text{mg}$$

16. Problem: 0.75 L   =   How many mL?
    Given quantity   =
    Wanted quantity   =

$$\frac{0.75\,L\quad|}{\qquad\qquad\qquad\qquad} = \quad \text{mL}$$

17. Problem: 3 hr   =   How many min?
    Given quantity   =
    Wanted quantity   =

$$\frac{3\,hr\quad|}{\qquad\qquad\qquad\qquad} = \quad \text{min}$$

18. Problem: 3.5 mL   =   How many M?
    Given quantity   =
    Wanted quantity   =

$$\frac{3.5\,mL\quad|}{\qquad\qquad\qquad\qquad} = \quad \text{M}$$

19. Problem: 500 mcg   =   How many mg?
    Given quantity   =
    Wanted quantity   =

$$\frac{500\,mcg\quad|}{\qquad\qquad\qquad\qquad} = \quad \text{mg}$$

20. Problem: 225 M   =   How many tsp?
    Given quantity   =
    Wanted quantity   =

$$\frac{225\,M\quad|}{\qquad\qquad\qquad\qquad} = \quad \text{tsp}$$

SUMMARY

Chapter 3 has introduced you to **dimensional analysis** with a step-by-step explanation and an opportunity to practice solving problems involving common equivalents.

ONE-FACTOR MEDICATION PROBLEMS

This chapter teaches you to interpret medication orders correctly and to calculate one-factor medication problems accurately using dimensional analysis. For accurate administration of medication, the "five rights of medication administration" form the foundation of communication between the physician and/or nurse practitioner and the nurse.

- The physician or nurse practitioner writes a medication order using the five rights.
- The nurse administers the medication to the patient based on the five rights.

To calculate the change from a one-factor–given quantity to a one-factor–wanted quantity using dimensional analysis, it is necessary to have a clear understanding of the five rights.

INTERPRETATION OF MEDICATION ORDERS

Physicians and nurse practitioners order medications utilizing the **five rights** of medication administration:

- Right **patient** (person receiving the medication)
- Right **drug** (name of the medication)
- Right **dosage** (amount of medication to be given)
- Right **route** (how the medication is to be given)
- Right **time** (when and how often the medication is to be given)

Once you are able to interpret the important components of an order for medication, you can perform accurate calculations for the correct medication dosage by using dimensional analysis.

EXAMPLE 4.1

In the following medication order, identify the five rights of medication administration.

Give gr 10 aspirin to Mrs. C. Clark orally every 4 hours as needed for fever.

Right **patient**	Mrs. C. Clark
Right **drug**	Aspirin/for fever
Right **dosage**	gr 10
Right **route**	orally (PO)
Right **time**	every 4 hrs as needed (PRN)

> **Practice Exercise 4.1** Five Rights of Medication Administration

Medication Order #1

Administer PO to Mr. S. Smith, Advil (ibuprofen) 400 mg every 6 hours for arthritis.

a. Right **patient**   _____

b. Right **drug**   _____

c. Right **dosage**   _____

d. Right **route**   _____

e. Right **time**   _____

Medication Order #2

Tylenol (acetaminophen) gr 10 PO every 4 hours for Mr. J. Jones PRN for headache.

a. Right **patient**   _____

b. Right **drug**   _____

c. Right **dosage**   _____

d. Right **route**   _____

e. Right **time**   _____

ONE-FACTOR MEDICATION PROBLEMS

Medication problems can be easily solved using the five steps of dimensional analysis:

- The first step in interpreting any physician's order for medication is to identify the **given quantity** or the exact dosage of medication that the physician has ordered.

- The second step is to identify the **wanted quantity** or the answer to the medication problem.
- The third step is to establish the **unit path** from the given quantity to the wanted quantity using equivalents as **conversion factors** to complete the problem. Identifying the dosage of medication available **(dose on hand)** is considered part of the unit path.
- The fourth step is to set up the problem to cancel out unwanted units.
- The fifth step is to multiply the numerators, multiply the denominators, and divide the product of the numerators by the product of the denominators to provide the numerical value of the wanted quantity or the answer to the problem.

You may choose to implement either the **sequential method** or the **random method** of dimensional analysis. The **sequential method** requires that conversion factors be factored into the unit path in a logical, sequential method to cancel out a preceding unit. The **random method** allows random placement of conversion factors within the unit path. The focus is on the correct placement of the conversion factor (dose on hand) in the unit path to correspond with the answer (wanted quantity). If the wanted quantity is tablets, then tablets must be in the numerator position in the unit path with the dosage in the denominator position. Below is an example of a one-factor problem showing the placement of components used in dimensional analysis.

Unit Path

Given Quantity	Conversion Factor for Given Quantity	Conversion Computation		Wanted Quantity
10 gr	tablets	10	=	2 tablets
	5 gr	5		
	Conversion Factor for Wanted Quantity			

EXAMPLE 4.2

The physician orders gr 10 aspirin orally every 4 hours as needed for fever. The unit dose of medication on hand is gr 5 per tablet (5 gr/tab). How many tablets will you administer?

Given quantity = 10 gr
Wanted quantity = tablets
Dose on hand = 5 gr/tab

Step 1: Identify the *given quantity* (the physician's order).

| 10 gr | |
|-------|---| =

Step 2: Identify the *wanted quantity* (the answer to the problem).

| 10 gr | |
|-------|---| = tablets

QUICK TIPS

10 gr is a numerator without a denominator and *tablets* is a numerator without a denominator. This is called a one-factor medication problem because the given quantity and the wanted quantity contain only numerators.

Step 3: Establish the *unit path* from the given quantity to the wanted quantity using equivalents as *conversion factors*.

| 10 gr | (tablets) | |
|-------|-----------|---| = tablets
| | 5 gr | |

QUICK TIPS

The dose on hand (5 gr/tablets) is an equivalent that is used as a conversion factor and factored into the unit path.

Step 4: Set up the problem to allow for cancellation of unwanted units.

| 10 ~~gr~~ | (tablets) | |
|-----------|-----------|---| = tablets
| | 5 ~~gr~~ | |

QUICK TIPS

The unwanted units (gr) can be canceled from the problem leaving the wanted quantity (tablets) in the numerator portion of the unit path that has been identified as the correct placement of the wanted quantity. The sequential method of dimensional analysis has been used to factor in (incorporate into the problem) the dose on hand which allows the previous unit (given quantity) to be canceled from the unit path. When using the sequential method of dimensional analysis, the conversion factor that is factored into the unit path always cancels out the preceding unit.

Step 5: Multiply the numerators, multiply the denominators, and divide the product of the numerators by the product of the denominators to provide the numerical value for the wanted quantity.

$$\frac{10 \ \cancel{gr} \ \left| \ \boxed{\text{tablets}} \ \right| \ 10}{\left| \ 5 \ \cancel{gr} \ \right| \ 5} = 2 \text{ tablets}$$

2 tablets is the wanted quantity and the answer to the problem.

EXAMPLE 4.3

Administer PO Advil (ibuprofen) 400 mg every 6 hours for arthritis. Dosage on hand is 200 mg/tablet. How many tablets will you give?

    Given quantity   = 400 mg
    Wanted quantity = tablets
    Dose on hand   = 200 mg/tablet

Step 1: Identify the *given quantity*.

$$\frac{400 \text{ mg}}{} \quad\quad\quad\quad\quad =$$

Step 2: Identify the *wanted quantity*.

$$\frac{400 \text{ mg}}{} \quad\quad\quad\quad\quad = \quad \text{tablets}$$

Step 3: Establish the unit path from the given quantity to the wanted quantity using equivalents as conversion factors.

$$\frac{400 \text{ mg}}{} \left| \frac{(\text{tablet})}{200 \text{ mg}} \right| = \text{ tablets}$$

Step 4: Set up the problem to allow for cancellation of unwanted units.

$$\frac{400 \text{ mg}}{} \left| \frac{(\text{tablet})}{200 \text{ mg}} \right| = \text{ tablets}$$

Step 5: Multiply the numerators, multiply the denominators, and divide the product of the numerators by the product of the denominators to provide the numerical value of the wanted quantity.

$$\frac{400 \text{ mg}}{} \left| \frac{(\text{tablet})}{200 \text{ mg}} \right| \frac{4}{2} = 2 \text{ tablets}$$

QUICK TIPS

The sequential method of dimensional analysis has been used to set up the problem. The unwanted units (mg) have been canceled from the unit path by correctly factoring in the dose on hand (200 mg/tablet). The same number of zeroes also has been canceled from the numerator and denominator portions of the unit path.

---

2 tablets is the wanted quantity and the answer to the problem.

EXAMPLE 4.4

Tylenol (acetaminophen) gr 10 PO every 4 hours for headache. The unit dose of medication on hand is 325 mg per caplet. How many caplets will you give?

    Given quantity   = 10 gr
    Wanted quantity = caplets
    Dose on hand   = 325 mg/caplet

Step 1: Identify the *given quantity*.

$$\frac{10 \text{ gr}}{} =$$

Step 2: Identify the *wanted quantity*.

$$\frac{10 \text{ gr}}{} = \text{caplets}$$

Step 3: Establish the unit path from the given quantity to the wanted quantity using equivalents as conversion factors.

$$\frac{10 \text{ gr}}{} \quad \frac{60 \text{ mg}}{1 \text{ gr}} \quad \frac{\text{(caplet)}}{325 \text{ mg}} = \text{caplets}$$

Step 4: Set up the problem to allow for cancellation of unwanted units.

$$\frac{10 \text{ gr}}{} \quad \frac{60 \text{ mg}}{1 \text{ gr}} \quad \frac{\text{(caplet)}}{325 \text{ mg}} = \text{caplets}$$

QUICK TIPS

The sequential method of dimensional analysis has been used to set up the problem. The unwanted unit (gr) has been canceled from the unit path by correctly factoring in a conversion factor (1 gr = 60 mg). The dose on hand (325 mg/caplet) is factored into the unit path that allows the unwanted unit (mg) to be canceled from the problem. The remaining unit (caplet) is in the numerator portion of the problem and correctly correlates with the wanted quantity in the numerator portion of the problem.

Step 5: Multiply the numerators, multiply the denominators, and divide the product of the numerators by the product of the denominators to provide the numerical value of the wanted quantity.

$$\frac{10 \text{ gr}}{} \quad \frac{60 \text{ mg}}{1 \text{ gr}} \quad \frac{\text{(caplet)}}{325 \text{ mg}} \quad \frac{10 \times 60}{1 \times 325} \quad \frac{600}{325} = 1.8 \text{ caplets}$$

1.8 caplets is the wanted quantity and the answer to the problem, but utilizing the "rounding off and up" rule, 2 caplets would be given.

QUICK TIPS

Dimensional analysis is a problem-solving method that uses critical thinking and is not a specific formula. Therefore, the important concept to remember is that ALL unwanted units must be canceled from the unit path. The random method of dimensional analysis also can be used when solving medication problems. When using the random method of dimensional analysis, the focus is on the correct placement of the conversion factor to correlate with the wanted quantity in the numerator portion of the unit path without regard to preceding units.

EXAMPLE 4.5

The random method of dimensional analysis will be used to calculate the answer for example 4.3.

Step 1: Identify the *given quantity*.

$$\frac{10 \text{ gr}}{} \quad \rule{4cm}{0.4pt} \quad =$$

Step 2: Identify the *wanted quantity*.

$$\frac{10 \text{ gr}}{} \quad \rule{4cm}{0.4pt} \quad = \quad \text{caplets}$$

Step 3: Establish the unit path from the given quantity to the wanted quantity using equivalents as conversion factors.

$$\frac{10 \text{ gr}}{} \quad \Big| \quad \frac{\text{(caplet)}}{325 \text{ mg}} \quad \Big| \quad \rule{2cm}{0.4pt} \quad = \quad \text{caplets}$$

QUICK TIPS

When using the random method of dimensional analysis, the focus is on the correct placement of the conversion factor in the unit path to correspond with the wanted quantity. The problem is set up correctly as long as the dose on hand (caplet) is in the numerator portion of the unit path to correlate with the wanted quantity (caplet) that also is in the numerator portion of the unit path.

Step 4: Set up the problem to allow for cancellation of unwanted units.

10 ~~gr~~	(caplet)	60 ~~mg~~	
	325 ~~mg~~	1 ~~gr~~	

$$= \text{caplets}$$

QUICK TIPS

A conversion factor (1 gr = 60 mg) is factored into the problem to cancel out the unwanted units (gr and mg) in the unit path. The remaining unit in the unit path (caplet) correctly correlates with the wanted quantity in the numerator portion of the problem.

Step 5: Multiply the numerators, multiply the denominators, and divide the product of the numerators by the product of the denominators to provide the numerical value of the wanted quantity.

10 ~~gr~~	(caplet)	60 ~~mg~~	10×60	600
	325 ~~mg~~	1 ~~gr~~	325×1	325

$$= 1.8 \text{ caplets}$$

1.8 caplets is the wanted quantity and the answer to the problem but utilizing the "rounding off and up" rule, 2 caplets would be given.

Practice Exercise 4.2   One-Factor Medication Problems

1. The physician orders BuSpar 7.5 mg PO TID for management of anxiety. The dosage of medication on hand is 5 mg per tablet.
   How many tablets will you give? _____

2. The physician orders Wellbutrin 100 mg PO BID for treatment of depression. The dosage of medication on hand is 50 mg per tablet.
   How many tablets will you give? _____

3. The physician orders Synthroid 0.075 mg PO daily for treatment of hypothyroidism. The dosage of medication on hand is 75 mcg per tablet.
   How many tablets will you give? _____

4. The physician orders Avandia 8 mg PO daily for control of type 2 diabetes mellitus. The dosage of medication on hand is 4 mg per tablet.
   How many tablets will you give? _____

5. The physician orders Lipitor 40 mg PO daily for management of hypercholesterolemia. The dosage of medication on hand is 80 mg per tablet.
   How many tablets will you give? _____

COMPONENTS OF A DRUG LABEL

All medications (stock and unit dose) are labeled with a drug label that includes specific information to assist in the accurate administration of the medication.
Information on the drug label includes:

- Name of the drug, including the trade name (name given by the pharmaceutical company identified with a trademark symbol) and the generic name (chemical name given to the drug)
- The dosage of medication (the amount of medication in each tablet, capsule, or liquid)
- The form of medication (tablet, capsule, or liquid)

- The expiration date (how long the medication will remain stable and safe to administer)
- The lot number (the batch series for the medication)
- The manufacturer (the pharmaceutical company that produced the medication)

Identifying the Components of Drug Labels

EXAMPLE 4.6

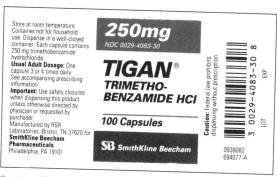

Courtesy of SmithKline Beecham Pharmaceuticals.

a. Trade name of the drug: Tigan
b. Generic name of the drug: Trimethobenzamide HCl
c. Dosage of medication: 250 mg per capsule
d. Form of medication: 100 capsules
e. Expiration date: Abbreviation display (number not listed)
f. Lot or batch number: Abbreviation displayed (number not listed)
g. Manufacturer: SmithKline Beecham

Practice Exercise 4.3　Identifying Components of a Drug Label

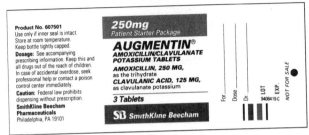

Courtesy of SmithKline Beecham Pharmaceuticals.

Augmentin

a. Trade name of the drug: _____
b. Generic name of the drug: _____
c. Dosage of medication: _____
d. Form of medication: _____
e. Expiration date: _____
f. Lot or batch number: _____
g. Manufacturer: _____

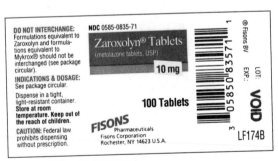

Courtesy of Fisons Pharmaceuticals.

Zaroxolyn

a. Trade name of the drug: _____
b. Generic name of the drug: _____

c. Dosage of medication: _____
d. Form of medication: _____
e. Expiration date: _____
f. Lot or batch number: _____
g. Manufacturer: _____

SOLVING PROBLEMS USING DRUG LABELS

Once you are able to identify the components of a drug label, you can use critical thinking to solve problems with dimensional analysis.

EXAMPLE 4.7

The physician orders Tegretol 200 mg PO BID as prophylaxis for tonic-clonic seizures. How many tablets will you give?

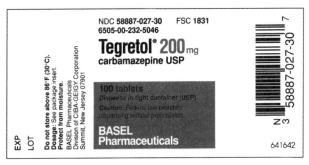

Courtesy of Basel Pharmaceuticals.

Given quantity   = 200 mg
Wanted quantity = tablets
Dose on hand   = 200 mg/tablet

Sequential method:

200 ~~mg~~	(tablet)	200	
	200 ~~mg~~	200	= 1 tablet

1 tablet is the wanted quantity and the answer to the problem.

EXAMPLE 4.8

The physician orders morphine 30 mg PO every 4 hours for management of severe pain. How many tablets will you give?

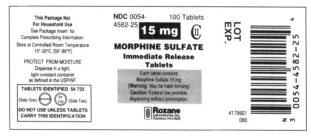

Courtesy of Roxane Laboratories Inc.

Given quantity   = 30 mg
Wanted quantity = tablets
Dose on hand   = 15 mg/tablet

Sequential method:

$$\frac{30 \ \cancel{mg} \quad | \quad \cancel{tablet} \quad | \quad 30}{15 \ \cancel{mg} \quad | \quad 15} = 2 \ \text{tablets}$$

2 tablets is the wanted quantity and answer to the problem.

EXAMPLE 4.9

The physician orders Detrol 2 mg PO daily for overactive bladder. How many tablets will you give?

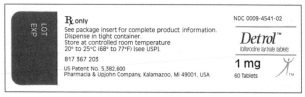

Courtesy of Pharmacia & Upjohn Company.

Given quantity   = 2 mg
Wanted quantity = tablets
Dose on hand   = 1 mg/tablet

Sequential method:

2 ~~mg~~	(tablet)	2	
	1 ~~mg~~	1	= 2 tablets

2 tablets is the wanted quantity and the answer to the problem.

Practice Exercise 4.4 Practice Problems with Drug Labels

1. The physician orders Lanoxin 0.25 mg PO once daily for 7 days for slow digitalization. How many tablets will you give? _____

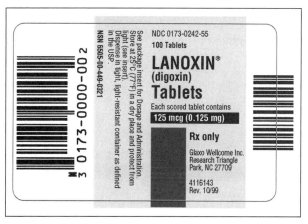

Courtesy of Glaxo Wellcome Inc.

(continued)

Practice Exercise 4.4   Practice Problems with
                            Drug Labels   (Continued)

2. The physician orders Tolinase 500 mg PO daily to
   control blood glucose. How many tablets will you
   give? _____

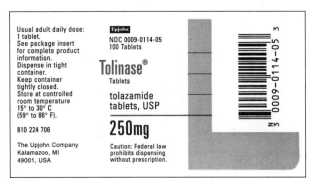

Usual adult daily dose:
1 tablet.
See package insert
for complete product
information.
Dispense in tight
container.
Keep container
tightly closed.
Store at controlled
room temperature
15° to 30° C
(59° to 86° F).

810 224 706

The Upjohn Company
Kalamazoo, MI
49001, USA

Upjohn
NDC 0009-0114-05
100 Tablets

Tolinase®
Tablets

tolazamide
tablets, USP

250mg

Caution: Federal law
prohibits dispensing
without prescription.

Courtesy of The Upjohn Company.

3. The physician orders Zaroxolyn 2.5 mg PO daily for
   management of mild hypertension. How many tablets
   will you give? _____

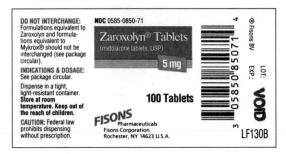

DO NOT INTERCHANGE:
Formulations equivalent to
Zaroxolyn and formula-
tions equivalent to
Mykrox® should not be
interchanged (see package
circular).

INDICATIONS & DOSAGE:
See package circular.

Dispense in a tight,
light-resistant container.
**Store at room
temperature. Keep out of
the reach of children.**

CAUTION: Federal law
prohibits dispensing
without prescription.

NDC 0585-0850-71

Zaroxolyn® Tablets
(metolazone tablets, USP)

5 mg

100 Tablets

FISONS
Pharmaceuticals
Fisons Corporation
Rochester, NY 14623 U.S.A.

LF130B

Courtesy of Fisons Pharmaceuticals.

4. The physician orders Zyban 150 mg PO BID for management of nicotine dependence. How many tablets will you give? _____

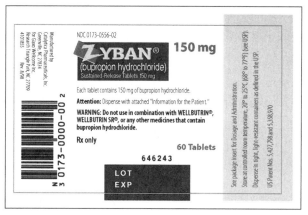

Courtesy of Glaxo Wellcome, Inc.

5. The physician orders Oramorph SR 30 mg PO every 4 hours PRN for management of severe pain. How many tablets will you give? _____

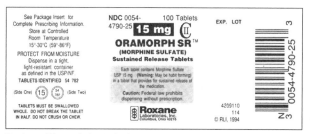

Courtesy of Roxane Laboratories Inc.

ADMINISTERING MEDICATION BY DIFFERENT ROUTES

Medication may be administered by a variety of different routes, including enteral or parenteral.

Enteral Medications

Oral (PO) medications are administered using tablets, caplets, capsules, or liquid.

- Tablets and caplets may be **scored,** which permits a more accurate administration when $\frac{1}{4}$ or $\frac{1}{2}$ of a tablet must be given.
- Tablets and caplets also may be **enteric coated,** allowing the medication to bypass disintegration in the stomach to decrease irritation and then break down in the small intestine for absorption. Enteric-coated tablets and caplets should never be crushed because the stomach would be irritated by the medication.
- Capsules are usually **time-released** and therefore should never be crushed or opened because the medication would be immediately released into the system instead of being released slowly over time.

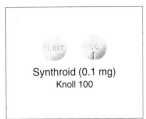

Synthroid (0.1 mg)
Knoll 100

Tablets: note scored tablet on right.

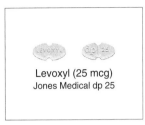

Levoxyl (25 mcg)
Jones Medical dp 25

Caplets: note scored caplet on right.

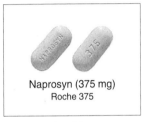

Naprosyn (375 mg)
Roche 375

Enteric coated caplets.

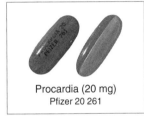

Procardia (20 mg)
Pfizer 20 261

Capsules.

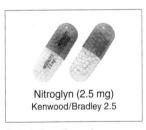

Nitroglyn (2.5 mg)
Kenwood/Bradley 2.5

Control released capsules.

- Liquid medication is accurately administered using a medication cup or medication syringe.
- The medication cup contains the common equivalents for the metric, apothecary, and household systems to permit adaptation of the medication's dosage for administration under various circumstances.

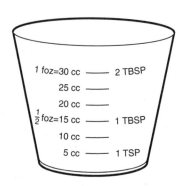

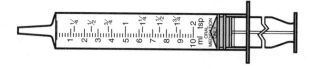

EXAMPLE 4.10

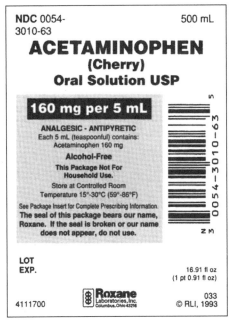

Courtesy of Roxane Laboratories, Inc.

Order: acetaminophen 320 mg PO every 4 hours for mild pain.
How many teaspoons will you give?

Given quantity   = 320 mg
Wanted quantity = tsp
Dose on hand   = 160 mg/5 mL

Sequential method:

32̶0̶ mg	5 mL̶	(tsp)	32 × 5	160	
16̶0̶ mg	5 mL̶	16 × 5	80	= 2 tsp

The wanted quantity and the answer to the problem is 2 tsp.

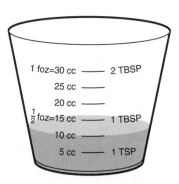

EXAMPLE 4.11

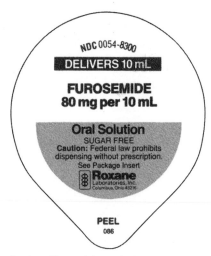

Courtesy of Roxane Laboratories Inc.

Order: furosemide 40 mg PO daily for management of congestive heart failure. How many milliliters will you give?

Given quantity   = 40 mg
Wanted quantity = mL
Dose on hand   = 80 mg/10 mL

Sequential method:

40 mg	10 mL	4 × 10	40	
	80 mg	8	8	= 5 mL

The wanted quantity and the answer to the problem is 5 mL.

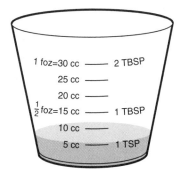

EXAMPLE 4.12

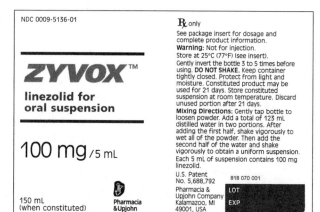

NDC 0009-5136-01

ZYVOX™

linezolid for
oral suspension

100 mg /5 mL

150 mL
(when constituted)

Pharmacia & Upjohn

R̸ only
See package insert for dosage and
complete product information.
Warning: Not for injection.
Store at 25°C (77°F) (see insert).
Gently invert the bottle 3 to 5 times before
using. **DO NOT SHAKE.** Keep container
tightly closed. Protect from light and
moisture. Constituted product may be
used for 21 days. Store constituted
suspension at room temperature. Discard
unused portion after 21 days.
Mixing Directions: Gently tap bottle to
loosen powder. Add a total of 123 mL
distilled water in two portions. After
adding the first half, shake vigorously to
wet all of the powder. Then add the
second half of the water and shake
vigorously to obtain a uniform suspension.
Each 5 mL of suspension contains 100 mg
linezolid.

U.S. Patent
No. 5,688,792   818 070 001

Pharmacia &
Upjohn Company
Kalamazoo, MI
49001, USA   LOT   EXP

Courtesy of Pharmacia & Upjohn Company.

Order: Zyvox 400 mg PO every 12 hours for skin infection. How many mL will you give?

Given quantity   = 400 mg
Wanted quantity = mL
Dose on hand   = 100 mg/5 mL

Sequential method:

$$\frac{400 \text{ mg}}{} \left| \frac{5 \text{ mL}}{100 \text{ mg}} \right| \frac{4 \times 5}{1} = 20 \text{ mL}$$

The wanted quantity and the answer to the problem is 20 mL.

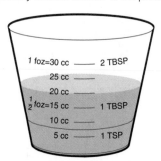

Practice Exercise 4.5 Administering Enteral Medications

1. Order: morphine sulfate 30 mg PO every 4 hours for management of severe pain. How many milliliters will you give? _____

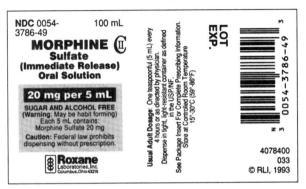

NDC 0054-3786-49   100 mL

MORPHINE (II)
Sulfate
(Immediate Release)
Oral Solution

20 mg per 5 mL

SUGAR AND ALCOHOL FREE
(Warning: May be habit forming)
Each 5 mL contains:
Morphine Sulfate 20 mg
Caution: Federal law prohibits
dispensing without prescription.

Roxane
Laboratories, Inc.
Columbus, Ohio 43216

Usual Adult Dosage: One teaspoonful (5 mL) every 4 hours or as directed by physician. Dispense in tight, light-resistant container as defined in the USP/NF. See Package Insert For Complete Prescribing Information. Store at Controlled Room Temperature 15°-30°C (59°-86°F)

LOT
EXP.

0054-3786-49

4078400
033
© RLI, 1993

Courtesy of Roxane Laboratories, Inc.

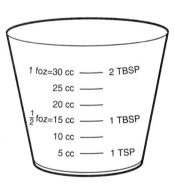

1 foz=30 cc ——— 2 TBSP
25 cc ———
20 cc ———
½ foz=15 cc ——— 1 TBSP
10 cc ———
5 cc ——— 1 TSP

(continued)

Practice Exercise 4.5 Administering Enteral
                        Medications (Continued)

2. Order: acetaminophen 325 mg every 4 hours for
   management of fever. How many milliliters will you
   give? _____

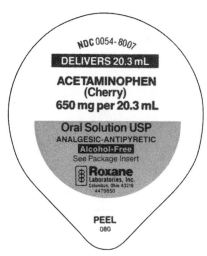

Courtesy of Roxane Laboratories, Inc.

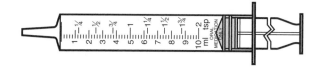

3. Order: lactulose 30 g PO QID for management of hepatic encephalopathy. How many milliliters will you give? _____

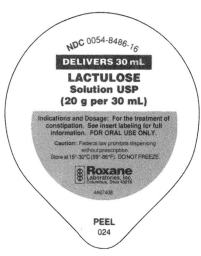

NDC 0054-8486-16

DELIVERS 30 mL

LACTULOSE
Solution USP
(20 g per 30 mL)

Indications and Dosage: For the treatment of constipation. See insert labeling for full information. FOR ORAL USE ONLY.

Caution: Federal law prohibits dispensing without prescription.
Store at 15°-30°C (59°-86°F). DO NOT FREEZE.

Roxane
Laboratories, Inc.
Columbus, Ohio 43216

4467408

PEEL
024

Courtesy of Roxane Laboratories, Inc.

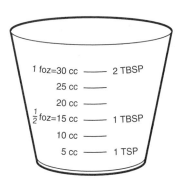

1 foz=30 cc —— 2 TBSP
25 cc ——
20 cc ——
½ foz=15 cc —— 1 TBSP
10 cc ——
5 cc —— 1 TSP

(continued)

Practice Exercise 4.5 Administering Enteral
Medications (Continued)

4. Order: ipecac syrup 15 mL PO to induce vomiting for
   management of overdose or poisoning. How many
   teaspoons will you give? _____

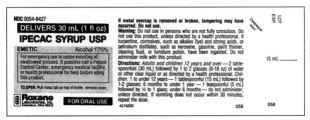

NDC 0054-8427

DELIVERS 30 mL (1 fl oz)

IPECAC SYRUP USP

EMETIC   Alcohol 1.75%

For emergency use to cause vomiting of
swallowed poisons. If possible call a Poison
Control Center, emergency medical facility,
or health professional for help before using
this product.

TO OPEN: Pull metal tab on top of bottle, remove cover.

Roxane
Laboratories, Inc.
Columbus, Ohio 43216   FOR ORAL USE

4216200

If metal overcap is removed or broken, tampering may have
occurred. Do not use.
Warning: Do not use in persons who are not fully conscious. Do
not use this product, unless directed by a health professional, if
turpentine, corrosives, such as alkalies (lye) and strong acids, or
petroleum distillates, such as kerosene, gasoline, paint thinner,
cleaning fluid, or furniture polish, have been ingested. Do not
administer milk with this product.
Directions: *Adults and children 12 years and over* — 2 table-
spoonfuls (30 mL) followed by 1 to 2 glasses (8-16 oz) of water
or other clear liquid or as directed by a health professional; *Children:* 1 to under 12 years — 1 tablespoonful (15 mL) followed by
1-2 glasses; 6 months to under 1 year — 1 teaspoonful (5 mL)
followed by ½ to 1 glass; under 6 months — do not administer,
unless directed. If vomiting does not occur within 30 minutes,
repeat the dose.

059   059

15 mL _____

LOT
EXP.

Courtesy of Roxane Laboratories, Inc.

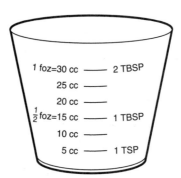

1 foz=30 cc ——— 2 TBSP

25 cc ———

20 cc ———

½ foz=15 cc ——— 1 TBSP

10 cc ———

5 cc ——— 1 TSP

5. Order: digoxin elixir 0.05 mg PO daily for congestive heart failure. How many milliliters will you give?

_____

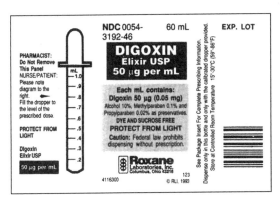

Courtesy of Roxane Laboratories, Inc.

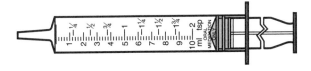

Parenteral Medications

Medications may also be ordered by the physician or nurse practitioner for the parenteral route of administration. Parenteral is defined as "by injection," including subcutaneous (SQ), intramuscular (IM), and intravenous (IV). Parenteral medications are sterile solutions obtained from vials or ampules and are administered using a syringe or prefilled syringes. The three syringes most often used are the **3-cc syringe, insulin syringe,** and **tuberculin syringe.**

3-cc Syringe

3-cc syringe (used for a variety of medications requiring administration of 0.2 to 3 cc).

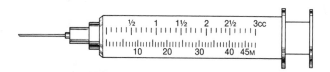

Insulin Syringe

Insulin syringe (used specifically to administer insulin). There are two types of insulin syringes that are graded in units, illustrated below.

- The U-100 insulin syringe is a 1-cc syringe with a 28-gauge ½-inch needle. The U-100 is a standard syringe that is graded with each mark equal to 2 units of insulin.

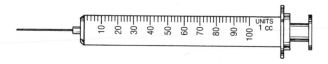

- The Lo-Dose insulin syringe is a ½-cc syringe with a 28-gauge ½-inch needle. The Lo-Dose is graded with each mark equal to 1 unit of insulin.

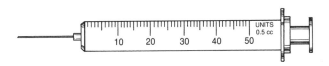

Tuberculin Syringe

Tuberculin syringe (used for a variety of medications requiring administration of doses from 0.1 to 1 cc). The tuberculin syringe is a 1-cc syringe with a 27-gauge ⅝-inch needle.

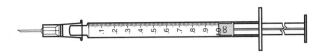

EXAMPLE 4.13

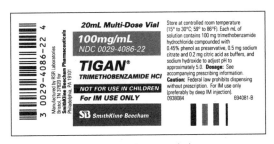

Courtesy of SmithKline Beecham Pharmaceuticals.

Order: Tigan 100 mg IM QID for nausea. How many mL will you give?

Given quantity   = 100 mg
Wanted quantity = mL
Dose on hand   = 100 mg/mL

Sequential method:

$$\frac{100 \text{ mg}}{} \Big| \frac{\text{mL}}{100 \text{ mg}} \Big| \frac{1}{1} = 1 \text{ mL}$$

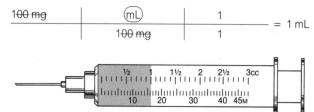

QUICK TIPS

Insulin is given with an insulin syringe that requires no calculation. The number of units of insulin ordered by the physician equals the number of units that the nurse draws up in the insulin syringe.

EXAMPLE 4.14

Order: Lente human insulin 45 units SQ every AM for type 1 diabetes mellitus. How many units will you give?

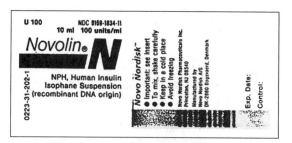

Courtesy of Novo Nordisk Pharmaceuticals Inc.

Sequential method:

$$45 \text{ units} \qquad\qquad = 45 \text{ units}$$

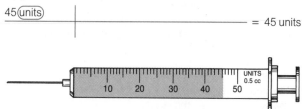

EXAMPLE 4.15

QUICK TIPS

When small amounts of medication need to be accurately administered, a tuberculin syringe is used because it is calibrated from 0.1 to 1 cc.

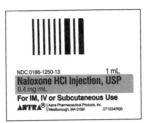

Courtesy of Astra Pharmaceutical Products, Inc.

Order: naloxone (Narcan) 40 mcg for opioid-induced respiratory depression with chronic use. How many milliliters will you give?

    Given quantity   = 40 mcg
    Wanted quantity = mL
    Dose on hand   = 0.4 mg/mL

Random method:

40 mcg	(mL)	1 mg	4 × 1	4	
	0.4 mg	1000 mcg	0.4 × 100	40	= 0.1 mL

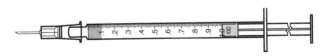

QUICK TIPS

Heparin is administered using a tuberculin syringe because the syringe is calibrated from 0.1 to 1 cc, allowing more accurate administration of doses smaller than 1 cc. Heparin can also be administered with prefilled heparin syringes.

EXAMPLE 4.16

Order: heparin 5000 units SQ BID for prevention of thrombi.

On hand: heparin 10,000 Units/mL

How many milliliters will you give?

Sequential method:

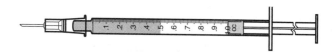

$$\frac{5000 \text{ units}}{} \quad \Big| \quad \frac{(\text{mL})}{10,000 \text{ units}} \quad \Big| \quad \frac{5}{10} \quad = 0.5 \text{ mL}$$

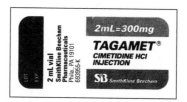

Practice Exercise 4.6   Parenteral Medications

1. Order: Tagamet 300 mg IM one hour before anesthesia to prevent aspiration pneumonitis. How many mL will you give? _____

2 mL vial
SmithKline Beecham
Pharmaceuticals
Phila., PA 19101
693955-K
LOT
EXP

2mL=300mg

TAGAMET®
CIMETIDINE HCl
INJECTION

SB *SmithKline Beecham*

Courtesy of SmithKline Beecham
Pharmaceuticals.

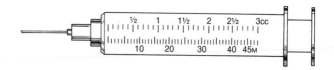

2. Order: magnesium sulfate 1000 mg IM every 6 hours for 4 hours over a 4-hr period. How many milliliters will you give? _____

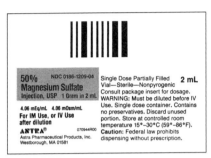

Courtesy of Astra Pharmaceutical Products, Inc.

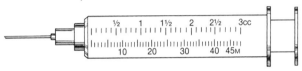

3. Order: Tigan 200 mg IM 3 to 4 times daily as needed for nausea and vomiting. How many milliliters will you give? _____

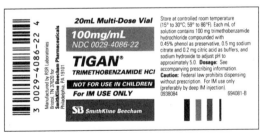

Courtesy of SmithKline Beecham Pharmaceuticals.

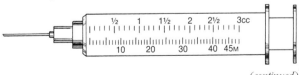

(continued)

Practice Exercise 4.6 Parenteral Medications (Continued)

4. Order: regular insulin 10 units SQ every AM for type 1 diabetes mellitus. On hand: Regular insulin 100 units/mL. How many units will you give? _____

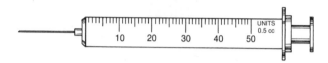

5. Order: heparin 5000 units SQ BID for prevention of thrombi. On hand: heparin 10,000 units/mL. How many milliliters will you give? _____

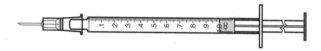

SUMMARY

Chapter 4 has helped you to interpret medication orders and drug labels correctly, and to calculate **one-factor-given quantity** to **one-factor-wanted quantity** medication problems accurately using the **sequential** or **random** problem-solving methods of dimensional analysis.

TWO-FACTOR MEDICATION PROBLEMS

This chapter will help you to accurately calculate medication problems using **dimensional analysis** that involve the **weight** of a patient, the **reconstitution** of medications from powder to liquid form, and the amount of **time** over which medications or intravenous fluids can be safely administered.

Although medications are ordered by physicians and/or nurse practitioners and administered by nurses using the "five rights of medication administration," other factors might need to be considered when administering certain medications or intravenous fluids.

- The **weight** of the patient often must be factored into a medication problem when determining how much medication can safely be given to an infant or a child.
- The dosage of medication available may be in a powdered form and need **reconstitution** to a liquid form prior to parenteral or intravenous administration.
- The length of **time** over which medications or intravenous fluids can be given plays an important role in the safe administration of intravenous therapy.

To be able to calculate **two-factor–given quantity** to **one-factor**–or **two-factor–wanted quantity** medication problems, it is important to understand all factors that may need consideration in some medication problems.

MEDICATION PROBLEMS INVOLVING WEIGHT

Using the five steps involved in problem solving with dimensional analysis, either the **sequential method** or the **random method** can be used to calculate two-factor–given quantity medication problems without difficulty.

- The **given quantity** (the physician's order) now contains two parts: a **numerator** (dosage of medication) and a **denominator** (the weight of the patient).
- This type of medication problem is called a **two-factor** medication problem because the given quantity now contains two parts (a numerator and a denominator) instead of just one part (a numerator).

EXAMPLE 5.1

The physician orders gentamicin 2.5 mg/kg IV (intravenous) every 8 hours for infection. The vial of medication is labeled 40 mg/mL. The child weighs 60 lb. How many milliliters will you give?

Given quantity   = 2.5 mg/kg
Wanted quantity = mL
Dose on hand   = 40 mg/mL
Weight   = 60 lb

QUICK TIPS

Identify the two-factor–given quantity (the physician's order) that contains two parts: a numerator (2.5 mg) and a denominator (kg). Identify the one-factor–wanted quantity (mL). Establish the unit path from the given quantity to the wanted quantity using equivalents as conversion factors.

Sequential method:

$$\frac{2.5 \text{ mg}}{\text{kg}} \quad\rule{6cm}{0.4pt}\quad = \quad \text{mL}$$

QUICK TIPS

The two-factor–given quantity has been set up correctly with a numerator (2.5 mg) and a denominator (kg) leading across the unit path to a one-factor–wanted quantity with only a numerator (mL).

$$\frac{2.5 \text{ mg}}{\text{kg}} \quad \frac{\text{(mL)}}{40 \text{ mg}} \quad\rule{4cm}{0.4pt}\quad = \quad \text{mL}$$

QUICK TIPS

The dose on hand (40 mg/mL) has been factored into the unit path to cancel out the preceding unwanted unit (mg). The wanted unit (mL) is in the numerator portion of the unit path and correctly corresponds with the one-factor–wanted quantity (mL).

2.5 mg	(mL)	1 kg		
kg	40 mg	2.2 lb	=	mL

QUICK TIPS

A conversion factor (1 kg = 2.2 lb) is now factored into the unit path to cancel out the preceding unwanted unit (kg).

2.5 mg	(mL)	1 kg	60 lb		
kg	40 mg	2.2 lb		=	mL

QUICK TIPS

The weight is finally factored into the unit path to cancel out the preceding unwanted unit (lb) in the denominator portion of the problem. All unwanted units are now canceled from the problem, and only the wanted unit (mL) remains in the numerator portion of the unit path, correctly corresponding with the one-factor–wanted quantity (mL). Multiply the numerators, multiply the denominators, and divide the product of the numerators by the product of the denominators to provide the numerical value for the one-factor–wanted quantity.

2.5 mg	(mL)	1 kg	60 lb	$2.5 \times 1 \times 6$	15	
kg	40 mg	2.2 lb		4×2.2	8.8	= 1.7 mL

1.7 mL is the wanted quantity and the answer to the problem.

Random method:

2.5 mg	1 kg	(mL)	60 lb	$2.5 \times 1 \times 6$	15	
kg	2.2 lb	40 mg		2.2×4	8.8	= 1.7 mL

Random method:

$$\frac{2.5 \text{ mg}}{\text{kg}} \mid \frac{1 \text{ kg}}{2.2 \text{ lb}} \mid \frac{60 \text{ lb}}{} \mid \frac{(\text{mL})}{40 \text{ mg}} \mid \frac{2.5 \times 1 \times 6}{2.2 \times 4} \mid \frac{15}{8.8} = 1.7 \text{ mL}$$

QUICK TIPS

Dimensional analysis is a problem-solving method that uses critical thinking. When implementing the random method of dimensional analysis, the medication problem can be set up in a number of different ways. The focus is on the correct placement of the conversion factors to cancel out all unwanted units. The wanted unit is placed in the numerator portion of the problem to correctly correspond with the wanted quantity.

Practice Exercise 5.1   **Involving Weight**

1. Order: Ceftin 15 mg/kg PO every 12 hr for pharyngitis tonsillitis. The patient weighs 110 lb. How many tablets will you give? _____

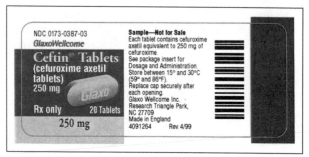

NDC 0173-0387-03
GlaxoWellcome
Ceftin® Tablets
(cefuroxime axetil
tablets)
250 mg
Glaxo
Rx only   20 Tablets
250 mg

Sample—Not for Sale
Each tablet contains cefuroxime
axetil equivalent to 250 mg of
cefuroxime.
See package insert for
Dosage and Administration.
Store between 15° and 30°C
(59° and 86°F).
Replace cap securely after
each opening.
Glaxo Wellcome Inc.
Research Triangle Park,
NC 27709
Made in England
4091264   Rev. 4/99

Courtesy of GlaxoWellcome.

2. Order: morphine sulfate 0.3 mg/kg PO for severe pain in opioid-naïve patient. The patient weighs 40 kg. How many milliliters will you give? _____

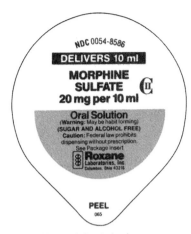

Courtesy of Roxane Laboratories, Inc.

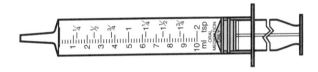

3. Order: Epogen 100 units/kg SQ three times weekly for 8 weeks for treatment of anemia secondary to AZT therapy. The patient weighs 100 lb. How many milliliters will you give? _____

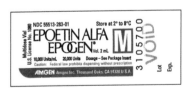

Courtesy of Amgen Inc.

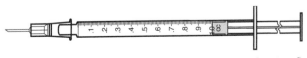

(continued)

Practice Exercise 5.1 Involving Weight (Continued)

4. Order: furosemide 1 mg/kg PO every 8 hours for congestive heart failure. The child weighs 20 kg. How many milliliters will you give? _____

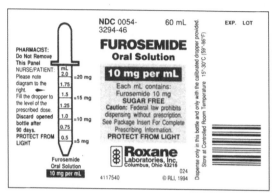

Courtesy of Roxane Laboratories, Inc.

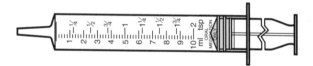

5. Order: Neupogen 6 mcg/kg SQ bid for severe chronic neutropenia. The patient weighs 50 kg. How many milliliters will you give? _____

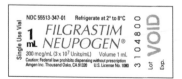

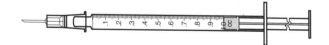

MEDICATION PROBLEMS INVOLVING RECONSTITUTION

Some medications in vials are in a powder form and need reconstitution before administration.

- **Reconstitution** involves adding a specific amount of sterile solution (also called **diluent**) to the vial to change the powder to a liquid form.
- Information as to how much diluent to add to the vial and what dosage of medication per milliliter will result after reconstitution (also called **yield**) can be obtained from a nursing drug reference, label, or package insert.

EXAMPLE 5.2

The physician orders Mezlin (mezlocillin) 50 mg/kg every 4 hours IV for infection. The child weighs 60 lb. The pharmacy sends a vial of medication labeled Mezlin 1 gram. The nursing drug reference provides information to reconstitute 1 gram of medication with 10 mL of sterile water for injection, 0.9% NaCl, or D5W. How many milliliters will you draw from the vial?

Given quantity   = 50 mg/kg
Wanted quantity = mL
Dose on hand   = 1 g/10 mL (yields 1 g/10 mL)
Weight   = 60 lb

Random method:

$$\frac{50\text{ mg}}{\text{kg}}\left|\frac{1\text{ kg}}{2.2\text{ lb}}\right|\frac{60\text{ lb}}{}\left|\frac{10\text{ mL}}{}\right|\frac{1\text{ g}}{}\left|\frac{1\text{ g}}{1000\text{ mg}}\right| \frac{5\times1\times6}{2.2} \frac{30}{2.2} = 13.63\text{ mL}$$

13.63 mL or 13.6 mL is the wanted quantity and the answer to the problem.

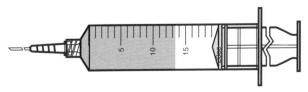

QUICK TIPS

A nursing drug reference, label, or package insert will provide information regarding how much and what type of diluent to use to reconstitute a drug, as well as what would be the yield or reconstitution. The five problem-solving steps of dimensional analysis remain applicable with any reconstitution medication problem.

Practice Exercise 5.2 Involving Reconstitution

1. The physician orders Zyvox (linezolid) 600 mg PO every 12 hours for infection associated with vancomycin-resistant *Enterococcus faecium*. The pharmacy sends a bottle of medication labeled Zyvox 150 mL. The label provides information to reconstitute with 123 mL of distilled water in two portions. How many milliliters will you pour from the bottle?

_____

NDC 0009-5136-01

℞ only

See package insert for dosage and complete product information.
Warning: Not for injection.
Store at 25°C (77°F) (see insert).
Gently invert the bottle 3 to 5 times before using. **DO NOT SHAKE.** Keep container tightly closed. Protect from light and moisture. Constituted product may be used for 21 days. Store constituted suspension at room temperature. Discard unused portion after 21 days.
Mixing Directions: Gently tap bottle to loosen powder. Add a total of 123 mL distilled water in two portions. After adding the first half, shake vigorously to wet all of the powder. Then add the second half of the water and shake vigorously to obtain a uniform suspension. Each 5 mL of suspension contains 100 mg linezolid.

ZYVOX™

linezolid for oral suspension

100 mg / 5 mL

150 mL (when constituted)

Pharmacia &Upjohn

U.S. Patent No. 5,688,792

818 070 001

Pharmacia & Upjohn Company Kalamazoo, MI 49001, USA

LOT

EXP

Courtesy of Pharmacia & Upjohn.

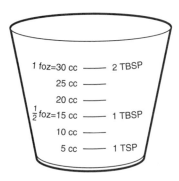

2. The physician orders Augmentin 12.5 mg/kg PO every 12 hours for otitis media. The child weighs 22 lb. The pharmacy sends a bottle of medication labeled Augmentin 75 mL. The label provides information to reconstitute with distilled water. How many milliliters will you pour from the bottle? _____

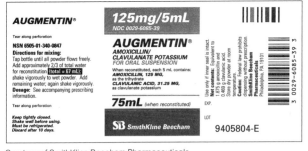

Courtesy of SmithKline Beecham Pharmaceuticals.

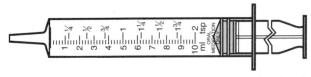

(continued)

Practice Exercise 5.2 Involving Reconstitution (Continued)

3. The physician orders Ancef 33.3 mg/kg IV 60 minutes before incision for perioperative prophylaxis and every 8 hours for 24 hours postoperative. The child weighs 50 lb. The pharmacy sends a vial of medication labeled Ancef 500 mg. The nursing drug reference provides information to reconstitute with 10 mL sodium chloride. How many milliliters will you draw from the vial? _____

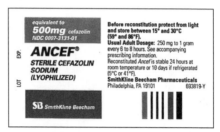

Courtesy of SmithKline Beecham Pharmaceuticals.

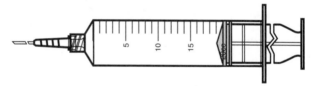

4. The physician orders Fortaz 50 mg/kg IV every 8 hours for meningitis. The child weighs 25 kg. The pharmacy sends a vial of medication labeled Fortaz 500 mg. The nursing drug reference provides information to reconstitute with 5 mL sodium chloride. How many milliliters will you draw from the vial? _____

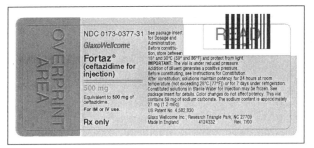

NDC 0173-0377-31

GlaxoWellcome

Fortaz®
(ceftazidime for
injection)

500 mg

Equivalent to 500 mg of
ceftazidime.

For IM or IV use.

Rx only

OVERPRINT AREA

See package insert
for Dosage and
Administration.
Before constitu-
tion, store between
15° and 30°C (59° and 86°F) and protect from light.
IMPORTANT: The vial is under reduced pressure.
Addition of diluent generates a positive pressure.
Before constituting, see Instructions for Constitution.
After constitution, solutions maintain potency for 24 hours at room
temperature (not exceeding 25°C (77°F)) or for 7 days under refrigeration.
Constituted solutions in Sterile Water for Injection may be frozen. See
package insert for details. Color changes do not affect potency. This vial
contains 59 mg of sodium carbonate. The sodium content is approximately
27 mg (1.2 mEq).

US Patent No. 4,582,830

Glaxo Wellcome Inc., Research Triangle Park, NC 27709
Made in England   4124332   Rev. 7/00

Courtesy of GlaxoWellcome.

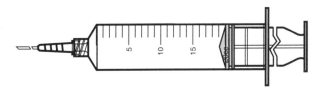

5. The physician orders vancomycin 7.5 mg/kg IV every
6 hours for osteomyelitis. The patient weighs 75 kg.
The pharmacy sends a vial of medication labeled vancomycin 500 mg. The nursing drug reference provides
information to reconstitute with 10 mL sodium chloride. How many milliliters will you draw from the vial?

_____

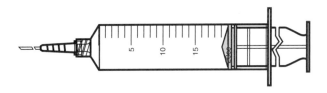

MEDICATION PROBLEMS INVOLVING INTRAVENOUS PUMPS

Intravenous medications are administered by drawing a specific amount of medication from a vial or ampule and inserting that medication into an existing intravenous line. All intravenous medications must be given with specific regard to exactly how much *time* it should take to administer the medication.

- Information regarding time may be obtained from a nursing drug reference, label, or package insert or may be specifically ordered by the physician.
- Although IV medications can be administered IV push, often the time involved requires the use of an intravenous pump (IV pump).
- All IV pumps deliver milliliters per hour (mL/hr or cc/hr) but may vary in operational capacity or size.

EXAMPLE 5.3

The physician orders heparin 1500 units/hr IV. The pharmacy sends an IV bag labeled: heparin 25,000 units in 250 mL of D5W. Calculate the number of milliliters per hour to set the IV pump.

    Given quantity   = 1500 units/hr
    Wanted quantity = mL/hr
    Dose on hand   = 25,000 units/250 mL

Begin by identifying the given quantity and establish the unit path to the wanted quantity.

Sequential method:

1500 units		mL
hr		hr

$$\frac{1500\ \text{units}}{\text{hr}} \quad \Bigg| \qquad\qquad\qquad = \quad \frac{\text{mL}}{\text{hr}}$$

QUICK TIPS

The two-factor–given quantity (the physician's order) contains two parts: a numerator (the dosage of medication) and a denominator (time). The wanted quantity (the answer to the problem) also contains two parts: a numerator (mL) and a denominator (time). This is called a two-factor–given quantity to a two-factor–wanted quantity medication problem. The denominator portion of the given quantity (hr) corresponds with the denominator portion of the wanted quantity (hr); therefore, only the numerator portion of the given quantity (units) needs to be canceled from the problem.

$$\frac{1500 \text{ units}}{\textcircled{hr}} \quad \Big| \quad \frac{250 \,\textcircled{mL}}{25,000 \text{ units}} \quad \Big| \quad \quad = \quad \frac{\text{mL}}{\text{hr}}$$

QUICK TIPS

After factoring the dose on hand into the unit path, the unwanted unit (units) is canceled from the problem and the wanted unit (mL) remains in the numerator portion of the problem to correspond with the wanted quantity. The same number of zeros and the same number values are canceled from the numerator and denominator portions of the problem, leaving 15 mL/hr as the wanted quantity and the answer to the problem.

$$\frac{1500 \text{ units}}{\textcircled{hr}} \quad \Big| \quad \frac{250 \,\textcircled{mL}}{25,000 \text{ units}} \quad \Big| \quad 15 \quad = \quad \frac{15 \text{ mL}}{\text{hr}}$$

EXAMPLE 5.4

The physician orders 500 mL of 0.45% NS with 20 mEq of KCl to infuse over 8 hours. Calculate the number of milliliters per hour to set the IV pump.

Given quantity   = 500 mL/8 hr
Wanted quantity = mL/hr

Sequential method:

$$\frac{500\ \text{(mL)}}{8\ \text{(hr)}} \quad \frac{500}{8} \quad = \quad \frac{62.5\ \text{mL}}{\text{hr}}\ \text{or}\ \frac{63\ \text{mL}}{\text{hr}}$$

63 mL/hr is the wanted quantity and the answer to the problem.

QUICK TIPS

In this problem the two factors needed for the wanted quantity are already identified in the given quantity and therefore require no additional conversions added to the unit path. The 20 mEq of KCl added to the IV bag is included as part of the 500 mL and is additional information for the nurse but not part of the calculation.

EXAMPLE 5.5

The physician orders aminophylline 44 mg/hr IV. The pharmacy sends an IV bag labeled: aminophylline 1 g/250 mL NS. Calculate the number of milliliters per hour to set the IV pump.

Given quantity   = 44 mg/hr
Wanted quantity = mL/hr
Dose on hand   = 1 g/250 mL

Random method:

$$\frac{44\ \cancel{\text{mg}}}{\text{(hr)}} \quad \frac{250\ \text{(mL)}}{1\ \cancel{\text{g}}} \quad \frac{1\ \cancel{\text{g}}}{1000\ \cancel{\text{mg}}} \quad \frac{44 \times 25}{100} \quad \frac{1100}{100} = \frac{11\ \text{mL}}{\text{hr}}$$

11 mL/hr is the wanted quantity and the answer to the problem.

QUICK TIPS

The given quantity has been identified as what the physician orders, but also can be information that the nurse has obtained. The nurse may know that the IV pump is set to deliver 11 mL/hr but wants to know if the dosage of medication that the patient is receiving is within a safe dosage range.

EXAMPLE 5.6

The nurse checks the IV pump and documents that the pump is set at and delivering 11 mL/hr and that the IV bag hanging is labeled: aminophylline 1 g/250 mL. How many milligrams per hour is the patient receiving?

Given quantity   = 11 mL/hr
Wanted quantity = mg/hr
Dose on hand   = 1 g/250 mL

Sequential method:

$$\frac{11 \text{ mL}}{\text{hr}} = \frac{\text{mg}}{\text{hr}}$$

QUICK TIPS

The given quantity is now identified as the information that the nurse has obtained and the wanted quantity is what the nurse would like to know.

$$\frac{11 \text{ mL}}{\text{hr}} \cdot \frac{1 \text{ g}}{250 \text{ mL}} = \frac{\text{mg}}{\text{hr}}$$

QUICK TIPS

The dose on hand is factored into the unit path, allowing the unwanted unit (mL) to be canceled from the problem.

$$\frac{11 \text{ mL}}{\text{hr}} \cdot \frac{1 \text{ g}}{250 \text{ mL}} \cdot \frac{1000 \text{ mg}}{1 \text{ g}} = \frac{11 \times 100}{25} = \frac{1100}{25} = \frac{44 \text{ mg}}{\text{hr}}$$

> ## QUICK TIPS
> Using the five steps of dimensional analysis, a variety of med-
> ication problems can be solved. Dimensional analysis is a
> critical thinking method that allows calculation of problems by
> identifying the given quantity (the physician's order or what
> the nurse knows) and establishing a unit path to the wanted
> quantity using the sequential method or the random method
> to solve one-factor or two-factor medication problems.

Practice Exercise 5.3 Involving Intravenous Pumps

1. The physician orders heparin 2500 units/hr IV for
   atrial fibrillation. The pharmacy sends an IV bag labeled: heparin 25,000 units in 250 mL of D5W.
   Calculate the number of milliliters per hour to set the
   IV pump. _____

2. The physician orders aminophylline 54 mg/hr IV for
   asthma. The pharmacy sends an IV bag labeled:
   aminophylline 1 g/250 mL NS. Calculate the number
   of milliliters per hour to set the IV pump. _____

3. The physician orders regular insulin 22 units/hr IV
   for ketoacidosis. The pharmacy sends an IV bag labeled: regulin insulin 100 units/100 mL normal saline.
   Calculate the number of milliliters per hour to set the
   IV pump. _____

4. The physician orders morphine 10 mg/hr continu-
   ous infusion for intractable pain. The pharmacy sends
   a 50 mL IV bag of normal saline labeled: morphine
   1 mg/mL. Calculate the number of milliliters per hour
   to set the IV pump. _____

5. The physician orders Dilaudid 20 mg/hr continu-
   ous infusion for severe pain. The pharmacy sends
   a 100 mL IV bag of normal saline labeled: Dilaudid
   2 mg/mL. Calculate the number of milliliters per hour
   to set the IV pump. _____

MEDICATION PROBLEMS INVOLVING DROP FACTORS

Although intravenous pumps are used whenever possible, there are situations (no IV pumps available) and circumstances (outpatient or home care) that arise when IV pumps are not available and IV fluids or medications might be administered using gravity flow.

- **Gravity flow** involves calculating the drops per minute (gtt/min) required to infuse IV fluids or medications.
- When IV fluids or medications are administered using **gravity flow,** it is important to know the **drop factor** for the IV tubing that is being used. **Drop factor** is the drops per milliliter (gtt/mL) that the IV tubing will produce.
- There are two types of IV tubing available for **gravity flow.**
  - **Macro** tubing delivers a large drop and is available in 10 gtt/mL, 15 gtt/mL, and 20 gtt/mL. **Table 5.1** summarizes different macrodrip factors.
  - **Micro** tubing delivers a small drop and is available in 60 gtt/mL.

Regardless of the IV tubing used, the five steps can be utilized and the problem can be solved using dimensional analysis as a problem-solving method.

● **Table 5.1 Examples of Different Macrodrip Factors**

MANUFACTURER	DROPS PER MILLILITER (GTT/ML)
Travenol	10
Abbott	15
McGaw	15
Cutter	20

EXAMPLE 5.7

The physician orders 250 mL of normal saline to infuse in 30 minutes. The drop factor listed on the IV tubing box is 10 gtt/mL. Calculate the drops per minute required to infuse the IV bolus.

Given quantity   = 250 mL/30 min
Wanted quantity = gtt/min
Drop factor   = 10 gtt/mL

QUICK TIPS

The given quantity and the wanted quantity both include two factors; therefore, this is a two-factor–given quantity to a two-factor–wanted quantity medication problem. Begin by identifying the given quantity and establish a unit path to the wanted quantity.

Sequential method:

$$\frac{250\ \text{mL}}{30\ \text{min}} \quad\bigg| \qquad\qquad = \quad \frac{\text{gtt}}{\text{min}}$$

QUICK TIPS

The denominators of the given quantity and the wanted quantity are the same (min). The numerator in the given quantity (mL) is an unwanted unit and needs to be canceled from the unit path.

$$\frac{250\ \text{mL}}{30\ \cancel{\text{min}}} \quad\bigg|\quad \frac{10\ \cancel{\text{gtt}}}{\text{mL}} \quad\bigg| \qquad\qquad = \quad \frac{\text{gtt}}{\text{min}}$$

QUICK TIPS

When the drop factor is factored into the unit path, the unwanted unit (mL) is canceled from the problem and the wanted unit (gtt) is correctly placed in the numerator portion of problem to correspond with the wanted quantity.

$$\frac{250 \text{ mL}}{30 \text{ min}} \left| \frac{10 \, \text{(gtt)}}{\text{mL}} \right| \frac{250 \times 1}{3} \left| \frac{250}{3} \right. = \frac{83.3 \text{ gtt}}{\text{min}} \text{ or } \frac{83 \text{ gtt}}{\text{min}}$$

QUICK TIPS

After the unwanted units are canceled from the problem, cancel the same number of zeros from the numerator and denominator portions of the problem, multiply the numerators, multiply the denominators, and divide the product of the numerators by the product of the denominators to provide the numerical value for the wanted quantity. 83 gtt/min is the wanted quantity and the answer to the problem.

EXAMPLE 5.8

The physician orders 1000 mL of D5W and 0.45% NS to infuse over 8 hours. The drop factor is 20 gtt/mL. Calculate the drops per minute required to infuse the IV volume.

Given quantity   = 1000 mL/8 hr
Wanted quantity = gtt/min
Drop factor   = 20 gtt/mL

Sequential method:

$$\frac{1000 \text{ mL}}{8 \text{ hr}} \left| \frac{20 \, \text{(gtt)}}{\text{mL}} \right| \qquad = \frac{\text{gtt}}{\text{min}}$$

QUICK TIPS

The unwanted unit (mL) is canceled from the problem and the wanted unit (gtt) is correctly placed in the numerator portion of the problem. Another unwanted unit (hr) needs to be canceled from the unit path.

$$\frac{1000 \text{ mL}}{8 \text{ hr}} \left| \frac{20 \, \text{(gtt)}}{\text{mL}} \right| \frac{1 \text{ hr}}{60 \, \text{(min)}} \qquad = \frac{\text{gtt}}{\text{min}}$$

QUICK TIPS

The conversion factor (1 hr = 60 min) has been factored into the problem to allow the unwanted unit (hr) to be canceled from the unit path and the wanted unit (min) is correctly placed in the denominator portion of the problem.

$$\frac{1000 \text{ mL}}{8 \text{ hr}} \left| \frac{20 \text{ (gtt)}}{\text{mL}} \right| \frac{1 \text{ hr}}{60 \text{ (min)}} \left| \frac{1000 \times 2 \times 1}{8 \times 6} \right| \frac{2000}{48} = \frac{41.66 \text{ gtt}}{\text{min}}$$

$$\frac{41.66 \text{ gtt}}{\text{min}} \quad \text{or} \quad \frac{42 \text{ gtt}}{\text{min}}$$

42 gtt/min is the wanted quantity and the answer to the problem.

QUICK TIPS

In some situations (home care), it may be important for the nurse to know exactly how long a specific amount of IV fluid will take to infuse. The physician may order a limited amount of IV fluid to infuse at a specific number of drops per minute.

EXAMPLE 5.9

The physician orders 1000 mL of D5W. The drop factor is 10 gtt/mL. The infusion is dripping at 21 gtt/min. How many hours will it take for the IV to infuse?

Given quantity   = 1000 mL
Wanted quantity = hr
Drop factor   = 10 gtt/mL

$$\frac{1000 \text{ mL}}{\rule{0pt}{2em}} \rule[-1em]{0.5pt}{2.5em} \hspace{6cm} = \qquad \text{hr}$$

QUICK TIPS

The given quantity and the wanted quantity have been identified and are both in the numerator portion of the problem; therefore, this is a one-factor–given quantity to a one-factor–wanted quantity medication problem.

$$\frac{1000 \text{ mL} \mid 10 \text{ gtt}}{\mid \text{mL}} = \text{hr}$$

QUICK TIPS

The drop factor (10 gtt/mL) has been factored into the problem using the sequential method to cancel the unwanted unit (mL) from the unit path.

$$\frac{1000 \text{ mL} \mid 10 \text{ gtt} \mid \text{min}}{\mid \text{mL} \mid 21 \text{ gtt}} = \text{hr}$$

QUICK TIPS

The infusing rate of 21 gtt/min has now been factored into the problem to cancel the unwanted unit (gtt) from the unit path.

$$\frac{1000 \text{ mL} \mid 10 \text{ gtt} \mid \text{min} \mid 1 \text{ hr}}{\mid \text{mL} \mid 21 \text{ gtt} \mid 60 \text{ min}} = \text{hr}$$

QUICK TIPS

The conversion factor (1 hr = 60 min) has been factored into the problem to cancel the unwanted unit (min) from the unit path. The wanted unit (hr) remains in the numerator portion of the problem that correctly corresponds with the wanted quantity.

$$\frac{1000 \text{ mL} \mid 10 \text{ gtt} \mid \text{min} \mid 1 \text{ hr}}{\mid \text{mL} \mid 21 \text{ gtt} \mid 60 \text{ min}} \quad \frac{1000 \times 1 \times 1}{21 \times 6} \quad \frac{1000}{126} = \frac{7.93 \text{ hr}}{\text{or 8 hr}}$$

QUICK TIPS

8 hr is the wanted quantity and the answer to the problem. It is safe nursing practice to monitor an infusing IV every 2 hours to make sure it is infusing without difficulty and on time. It may be necessary to hang the next IV after 7½ hr (before the estimated completion time) to keep the IV from running dry.

Practice Exercise 5.4 Involving Drop Factors

1. Order: Infuse 1000 mL D5W over 12 hours.
   Drop factor: 20 gtt/mL
   Calculate the number of drops per minute. _____
2. Order: Infuse 250 mL normal saline over 30 minutes.
   Drop factor: 10 gtt/mL
   Calculate the number of drops per minute. _____
3. Order: 1000 mL of D5W/0.9% NS.
   Drop factor: 20 gtt/mL
   Infusion rate: 50 gtt/min
   Calculate the number of hours to infuse. _____
4. Order: 500 mL lipids over 8 hours.
   Drop factor: 10 gtt/mL
   Calculate the number of drops per minute. _____
5. Infuse 1000 mL D5W at 150 mL/hr.
   Drop factor: 20 gtt/mL
   Calculate the number of drops per minute. _____

MEDICATION PROBLEMS INVOLVING INTERMITTENT INFUSION

Intravenous medications can be delivered over a specific amount of time by *intermittent infusion*.

- When medications are delivered by intermittent infusion, they require the use of an infusion pump.
- Some medications must be reconstituted and further diluted in a specific type and amount of IV fluid and delivered over a limited amount of time.
- Other medications do not need to be reconstituted but must be further diluted in a specific type and amount of IV fluid and delivered over a limited amount of time.

EXAMPLE 5.10

The physician ordered erythromycin 500 mg IV every 6 hr for infection. The pharmacy sends a vial labeled: erythromycin 1 g.

The nursing drug reference provides information to reconstitute 1 g of erythromycin with 20 mL of sterile water and further dilute in 250 mL of 0.9% NS, then infuse over 1 hour. How many milliliters will you draw from the vial after reconstitution? Calculate the number of milliliters per hour to set the IV pump.

QUICK TIPS

This order really contains two problems. The first problem involves deciding how many milliliters to draw from the vial after reconstitution and the second problem involves how many milliliters per hour to set the IV pump. Calculate each part of the problem using dimensional analysis as a problem-solving method.

How many mL will you draw from the vial after reconstitution?

Given quantity   = 500 mg
Wanted quantity = mL
Dose on hand   = 1 g/20 mL

Random method:

$$\frac{500 \text{ mg}}{} \left| \frac{20 \text{ mL}}{1 \text{ g}} \right| \frac{1 \text{ g}}{1000 \text{ mg}} \left| \frac{5 \times 2}{1} \right| \frac{10}{1} = 10 \text{ mL}$$

QUICK TIPS

10 mL is the wanted quantity and the amount that will need to be drawn from the vial and added to the 250 mL of 0.9% NS. After adding the 10 mL to the IV bag, the IV bag will now contain 260 mL.

Calculate the number of milliliters per hour to set the IV pump.

Given quantity   = 260 mL/1 hr
Wanted quantity = mL/hr

Sequential method:

$$\frac{260 \text{ mL}}{1 \text{ hr}} \left| \frac{260}{1} \right. = \frac{260 \text{ mL}}{\text{hr}}$$

The IV pump is set at 260 mL/hr to infuse the 500 mg of eryth-romycin ordered by the physician.

If an IV pump was unavailable, the infusion could be deliv-ered by gravity using IV tubing with a drop factor of 10 gtt/mL.

Calculate the gtt/min required to infuse the IV volume.

Given quantity   = 260 mL/1 hr
Wanted quantity = gtt/min
Drop factor   = 10 gtt/mL

Sequential method:

260 mL	10 gtt	1 hr	260 × 1	260		43.3 or 43 gtt
1 hr	mL	60 min	6	6	=	min

Practice Exercise 5.5 Involving Intermittent Infusion

1. Order: Ancef 500 mg IV every 8 hours for septicemia.
   Supply: Ancef 1 g vial
   Nursing drug reference: Reconstitute with 10 mL if 0.9% NS and further dilute in 100 mL NS. Infuse over 60 minutes.
   How many milliliters will you draw from the vial after reconstitution? _____
   Calculate the number of milliliters per hour to set the IV pump. _____
   Calculate the number of drops per minute with a drop factor of 20 gtt/mL. _____
2. Order: Fortaz 1 g IV every 8 hours for respiratory tract infection.
   Supply: Fortaz 1-g vial
   Nursing drug reference: Reconstitute with 10 mL of sodium chloride and further dilute in 100 mL NS. Infuse over 60 minutes.
   How many milliliters will you draw from the vial after reconstitution? _____
   Calculate the number of milliliters per hour to set the IV pump. _____

Calculate the number of drops per minute with a drop factor of 20 gtt/mL. _____

3. Order: vancomycin 500 mg every 8 hours for endo-carditis.

Supply: vancomycin 1-g vial

Nursing drug reference: Reconstitute with 10 mL sodium chloride and further dilute in 200 mL. Infuse over 60 minutes.

How many milliliters will you draw from the vial after reconstitution? _____

Calculate the number of milliliters per hour to set the IV pump. _____

Calculate the number of drops per minute with a drop factor of 20 gtt/mL. _____

4. Order: Cleocin 300 mg IV every 6 hours for treat-ment of skin infection.

Supply: Cleocin 600 mL/4-mL vial

Nursing drug reference: Further dilute in 50 mL D5W and infuse over 20 minutes.

How many milliliters will you draw from the vial after reconstitution? _____

Calculate the number of milliliters per hour to set the IV pump. _____

Calculate the number of drops per minute with a drop factor of 20 gtt/mL. _____

5. Order: Mezlin 3 g IV every 6 hours for urinary tract infection.

Supply: Mezlin 3-g vial

Nursing drug reference: Reconstitute with 10 mL D5W and further dilute in 100 mL D5W. Infuse over 30 minutes.

How many milliliters will you draw from the vial after reconstitution? _____

Calculate the number of milliliters per hour to set the IV pump. _____

Calculate the number of drops per minute with a drop factor of 20 gtt/mL. _____

SUMMARY

Chapter 5 has helped you to calculate **two-factor** medication problems involving the **weight** of the patient, **reconstitution** of medications, and the amount of **time** over which medications and intravenous fluids can be safely administered using the sequential or random method of dimensional analysis.

THREE-FACTOR MEDICATION PROBLEMS

This chapter will help you to accurately calculate medication problems involving the dosage of medication based upon the weight of the patient and the time required for safe administration using dimensional analysis as a problem-solving method.

- When medications are ordered by physicians or nurse practitioners for infants and children, the dosage of medication (g, mg, mcg, gr) based upon the weight of the child must be considered as well as how much medication the child can receive per dose or day. Although the physician orders the medications, the nurse must be aware of the **safe dosage range** for administration of medications to infants and children as well as critically ill adults.

- When medications are ordered by physicians for critically ill patients, the patients must be closely monitored by the nurse for effectiveness of the medications. Often the medications or intravenous fluids must be titrated for effectiveness with an increase or decrease in the dosage based upon the patient's response to the medications. Factors involved in the safe administration of medications or intravenous fluids for the critically ill patient include the dosage of medication based upon the combined factors of the weight of the patient and the time required for administration. The medication may need reconstitution or preparation by the nurse for immediate administration in a critical situation. The weight of the patient also may need to be obtained daily to ensure accurate correlation with the dosage of medication ordered.

To be able to calculate three-factor–given quantity to one-factor–, two-factor–, or three-factor–wanted quantity medication problems, it is necessary to understand all of the components of the medication order and be able to calculate medication problems in a critical situation.

MEDICATION PROBLEMS INVOLVING DOSAGE, WEIGHT, AND TIME

Utilizing the five problem-solving steps, three-factor–given quantity medication problems can be solved by implementing the sequential method or the random method of dimensional analysis. The given quantity (the physician's order) now contains three parts: a numerator (the dosage of medication ordered) and two denominators (the weight of the patient and the time required for safe administration).

EXAMPLE 6.1

The physician orders Tagamet 30 mg/kg/day PO in four divided doses for GI ulcers in a child weighing 22 kg. The dose on hand is Tagamet 300 mg/5 mL. How many milliliters per day will the child receive?

Given quantity	=	30 mg/kg/day
Wanted quantity	=	mL/day
Dose on hand	=	300 mg/5 mL
Weight	=	22 kg

QUICK TIPS

Identify the three-factor–given quantity (the physician's order) that contains three parts: a numerator (30 mg) and two denominators (kg/day). Establish the unit path from the given quantity (30 mg/kg/day) to the two-factor–wanted quantity (mL/day) utilizing the sequential method of dimensional analysis and the necessary conversion factors.

Sequential method:

$$\frac{30 \text{ mg}}{\text{kg/day}} \bigg| \hspace{6cm} = \frac{\text{mL}}{\text{day}}$$

QUICK TIPS

The three-factor–given quantity has been set up correctly with a numerator (30 mg) and two denominators (kg/day) leading across the unit path to a two-factor–wanted quantity with a numerator (mL) and a denominator (day). The conversion factors can now be factored into the unit path to allow cancellation of unwanted units.

$$\frac{30 \text{ mg}}{\text{kg/\cancel{day}}} \bigg| \frac{5 \text{ mL}}{300 \text{ mg}} \bigg| \hspace{4cm} = \frac{\text{mL}}{\text{day}}$$

QUICK TIPS

The dose on hand (300 mg/5 mL) has been factored into the unit path and correctly placed so that the wanted unit (mL) correlates with the wanted quantity (mL) and the unwanted unit (mg) is canceled from the problem.

$$\frac{30 \text{ mg}}{\text{kg/\cancel{day}}} \bigg| \frac{5 \text{ mL}}{300 \text{ mg}} \bigg| 22 \text{ kg} \hspace{3cm} = \frac{\text{mL}}{\text{day}}$$

QUICK TIPS

The weight of the child (22 kg) has been factored into the unit path and set up correctly to allow the unwanted unit (kg) to be canceled from the problem.

$$\frac{30 \text{ mg}}{\text{kg/\cancel{day}}} \bigg| \frac{5 \text{ mL}}{300 \text{ mg}} \bigg| 22 \text{ kg} \bigg| \frac{3 \times 5 \times 22}{30} \bigg| \frac{330}{30} = \frac{11 \text{ mL}}{\text{day}}$$

QUICK TIPS

All the unwanted units have been canceled from the unit path and the wanted units are correctly placed to correlate with the two-factor–wanted quantity (mL/day). Multiply numerators, multiply denominators, and divide the product of the numerators by the product of the denominators to provide the numerical answer to the problem. The wanted quantity is 11 mL/day.

Using dimensional analysis, calculate how many milliliters per dose the child should receive.

Given quantity	=	11 mL/day
Wanted quantity	=	mL/dose

$$\frac{11 \text{ mL}}{\text{day}} \quad\Bigg| \qquad\qquad\qquad = \qquad \frac{\text{mL}}{\text{dose}}$$

QUICK TIPS

The child is to receive 11 mL/day in four divided doses; therefore, the conversion factor involves how many doses are in a day (4 divided doses = day).

$$\frac{11 \;\cancel{(\text{mL})}}{\cancel{\text{day}}} \quad\Bigg|\quad \frac{\cancel{\text{day}}}{4 \;\cancel{(\text{doses})}} \quad\Bigg|\quad \frac{11}{4} = \frac{2.75 \text{ or } 2.8 \text{ mL}}{\text{dose}}$$

The wanted quantity is 2.8 mL/dose, and the child will receive this orally (PO) four times a day (QID).

The problem could have been set up to find the wanted quantity of mL/dose.

Given quantity	=	30 mg/kg/day
Wanted quantity	=	mL/dose
Dose on hand	=	300 mg/5 mL
Weight	=	22 kg

Sequential method:

$$\frac{30\ \text{mg}}{\text{kg/day}}\bigg|\frac{5\ \textcircled{mL}}{300\ \text{mg}}\bigg|\frac{22\ \text{kg}}{}\bigg|\frac{\text{day}}{4\ \textcircled{doses}}\bigg|\frac{3\times5\times22}{30\times4}\bigg|\frac{330}{120}=\frac{2.75\ \text{or}\ 2.8\ \text{mL}}{\text{dose}}$$

The wanted quantity is 2.8 mL/dose, and the child will receive this orally (PO) four times a day (QID).

EXAMPLE 6.2

As a prudent nurse, you are concerned that the child may be receiving an unsafe dosage of Tagamet; therefore, you want to identify how many mg/kg/day the child weighing 22 kg is receiving. The dosage of medication being given four times a day is 2.8 mL/dose. The dosage on hand is 300 mg/5 mL. How many milligrams per kilogram per day is the child receiving?

Given quantity	=	2.8 mL/dose
Wanted quantity	=	mg/kg/dose
Dose on hand	=	300 mg/5 mL
Weight	=	22 kg

Sequential method:

$$\frac{2.8\ \text{mL}}{\text{dose}}\bigg|=\frac{\text{mg}}{\text{kg/day}}$$

> ### QUICK TIPS
> The two-factor–given quantity (2.8 mL/dose) has been correctly factored into the unit path with a numerator (2.8 mL) and a denominator (dose). The three-factor–wanted quantity (mg/kg/day) also has been correctly factored into the unit path with a numerator (mg) and two denominators (kg/day).

$$\frac{2.8\ \text{mL}}{\text{dose}}\bigg|\frac{300\ \textcircled{mg}}{5\ \text{mL}}\bigg|\frac{4\ \text{doses}}{\text{day}}\bigg|\frac{}{22\ \text{kg}}=\frac{\text{mg}}{\text{kg/day}}$$

QUICK TIPS

The conversion factors have been added to the unit path and all unwanted units have been canceled from the problem. The wanted unit (mg) is correctly placed in the numerator portion of the problem to correlate with the wanted quantity (mg) also in the numerator portion of the three-factor–wanted quantity. The wanted units (kg and day) are in the denominator portion of the problem to correlate with the wanted quantity (kg and day) in the denominator portion of the three-factor–wanted quantity.

$$\frac{2.8 \text{ mL}}{\text{dose}} \left| \frac{300 \text{ mg}}{5 \text{ mL}} \right| \frac{4 \text{ doses}}{\text{day}} \left| \frac{}{22 \text{ kg}} \right| \quad \frac{2.8 \times 300 \times 4}{5 \times 22} = \frac{3360}{110} = \frac{30.54 \text{ mg}}{\text{kg/day}}$$

or $\dfrac{30.5 \text{ mg}}{\text{kg/day}}$

The three-factor–wanted quantity is 30.5 mg/kg/day.

QUICK TIPS

The nursing drug reference identifies that 20 to 40 mg/kg/day in four divided doses is a safe dosage of Tagamet for children. Therefore, the nurse is assured that the child is receiving a correct dosage. Dimensional analysis helps you to critically think through any type of medication problem.

EXAMPLE 6.3

The physician orders dobutamine 5 mcg/kg/min IV for cardiac failure. The pharmacy sends an IV bag labeled: dobutamine 250 mg/50 mL D5W/0.45% NS. The patient weighs 165 lb. Calculate the number of milliliters per hour to set the IV pump.

Given quantity	=	5 mcg/kg/min
Wanted quantity	=	mL/hr
Dose on hand	=	250 mg/50 mL
Weight	=	165 lb

QUICK TIPS

Identify the three-factor–given quantity (the physician's order) containing three parts: the numerator (5 mg) and two denominators (kg/min). Establish the unit path from the three-factor–given quantity to the two-factor–wanted quantity (mL/hr).

Random method:

$$\frac{5\ mcg}{kg/min}\ \bigg|\hspace{4cm}=\ \frac{mL}{hr}$$

QUICK TIPS

The three-factor–given quantity has been set up correctly with a numerator (5 mg) and two denominators (kg/min) leading across the unit path to a two-factor–wanted quantity with a numerator (mL) and a denominator (hr). Utilizing the random method of dimensional analysis, the conversion factors are factored into the unit path to cancel out unwanted units.

$$\frac{5\ mcg}{kg/\cancel{min}}\ \bigg|\ \frac{60\ \cancel{min}}{1\ \textcircled{hr}}\ \bigg|\hspace{3cm}=\ \frac{mL}{hr}$$

QUICK TIPS

The unwanted unit (min) has been canceled from the unit path by factoring the conversion factor (1 hr = 60 min), and the wanted unit correctly corresponds with the wanted quantity denominator (hr).

$$\frac{5\ mcg}{kg/\cancel{min}}\ \bigg|\ \frac{60\ \cancel{min}}{1\ \textcircled{hr}}\ \bigg|\ \frac{50\ \textcircled{mL}}{250\ mg}\hspace{1.5cm}=\ \frac{mL}{hr}$$

QUICK TIPS

The dose on hand (250 mg/50 mL) has been factored into the unit path and placed so that the wanted unit (mL) correctly corresponds with the wanted quantity numerator (mL).

$$\frac{5 \text{ mcg}}{\text{kg/min}} \left| \frac{60 \text{ min}}{1 \text{ hr}} \right| \frac{50 \text{ mL}}{250 \text{ mg}} \left| \frac{1 \text{ mg}}{1000 \text{ mcg}} \right. = \frac{\text{mL}}{\text{hr}}$$

QUICK TIPS

The conversion factor (1 mg = 1000 mcg) has been factored into the unit path to cancel the unwanted units (mg and mcg).

$$\frac{5 \text{ mcg}}{\text{kg/min}} \left| \frac{60 \text{ min}}{1 \text{ hr}} \right| \frac{50 \text{ mL}}{250 \text{ mg}} \left| \frac{1 \text{ mg}}{1000 \text{ mcg}} \right| \frac{1 \text{ kg}}{2.2 \text{ lb}} \left| 165 \text{ lb} \right. = \frac{\text{mL}}{\text{hr}}$$

QUICK TIPS

The final conversion factors (1 kg = 2.2 lb) and the weight of the patient have been factored into the unit path to cancel the remaining unwanted units (kg and lb). All the unwanted units have been canceled from the unit path and the wanted units (mL and hr) remain in the unit path in the correct positions to correlate with the two-factor–wanted quantity (mL/hr). Multiply the numerators, multiply the denominators, and divide the product of the numerators by the product of the denominators to provide the numerical value for the two-factor–wanted quantity.

$$\frac{5 \text{ mcg}}{\text{kg/min}} \left| \frac{60 \text{ min}}{1 \text{ hr}} \right| \frac{50 \text{ mL}}{250 \text{ mg}} \left| \frac{1 \text{ mg}}{1000 \text{ mcg}} \right| \frac{1 \text{ kg}}{2.2 \text{ lb}} \left| 165 \text{ lb} \right. = \frac{\text{mL}}{\text{hr}}$$

$$\frac{5 \times 6 \times 5 \times 1 \times 165}{25 \times 100 \times 2.2} \left| \frac{24750}{5500} \right. = \frac{4.5 \text{ mL}}{\text{hr}}$$

QUICK TIPS

4.5 mL/hr is the wanted quantity and the answer to the problem. IV pumps used in critical care can be set to deliver amounts including decimal points, so it is not necessary to round up the answer.

EXAMPLE 6.4

The nurse has been monitoring the hemodynamic readings of a patient weighing 165 lb receiving dobutamine 250 mg in 50 mL of D5W/0.45% NS and has received additional orders from the physician to titrate for effectiveness. The IV pump is now set at 9 mL/hr and the physician wants to know how many micrograms per kilogram per minute the patient is now receiving.

Given quantity	=	9 mL/hr
Wanted quantity	=	mcg/kg/min
Dose on hand	=	250 mg/50 mL
Weight	=	165 lb

$$\frac{9 \text{ mL}}{\text{hr}} \Bigg| \rule{4cm}{0pt} = \frac{\text{mcg}}{\text{kg/min}}$$

QUICK TIPS

The two-factor–given quantity is identified as the information that the nurse obtained from the IV pump and the three-factor–wanted quantity is the information that the physician has requested.

Sequential Method:

$$\frac{9 \text{ mL}}{\text{hr}} \Bigg| \frac{250 \text{ mg}}{50 \text{ mL}} = \frac{\text{mcg}}{\text{kg/min}}$$

QUICK TIPS

The dose on hand (the IV fluid that is presently infusing) has been factored into the unit path to cancel the unwanted unit (mL) from the problem.

$$\frac{9 \text{ mL}}{\text{hr}} \left| \frac{250 \text{ mg}}{50 \text{ mL}} \right| \frac{1000 \text{ mcg}}{1 \text{ mg}} = \frac{\text{mcg}}{\text{kg/min}}$$

QUICK TIPS

The conversion factor (1 mg = 1000 mcg) has been factored into the unit path to cancel the unwanted unit (mg) from the problem. The wanted unit (mcg) remains in the unit path and correctly corresponds with the wanted quantity in the numerator portion of the problem.

$$\frac{9 \text{ mL}}{\text{hr}} \left| \frac{250 \text{ mg}}{50 \text{ mL}} \right| \frac{1000 \text{ mcg}}{1 \text{ mg}} \left| \frac{1 \text{ hr}}{60 \text{ min}} \right. = \frac{\text{mcg}}{\text{kg/min}}$$

QUICK TIPS

The conversion factor (1 hr = 60 min) has been factored into the unit path to cancel the unwanted unit (hr) from the problem. The wanted unit (min) remains in the unit path, correctly placed in the denominator portion of the problem.

$$\frac{9 \text{ mL}}{\text{hr}} \left| \frac{250 \text{ mg}}{50 \text{ mL}} \right| \frac{1000 \text{ mcg}}{1 \text{ mg}} \left| \frac{1 \text{ hr}}{60 \text{ min}} \right| \frac{2.2 \text{ lb}}{1 \text{ kg}} \left| \frac{}{165 \text{ lb}} \right. = \frac{\text{mcg}}{\text{kg/min}}$$

QUICK TIPS

The conversion factor (1 kg = 2.2 lb) has been factored into the unit path to correspond with the wanted quantity denominator (kg). The weight of the patient also is factored into the unit path to cancel the unwanted unit (lb) from the problem. After all unwanted units have been canceled from the problem and the wanted units correctly identified, multiply the numerators, multiply the denominators, and divide the product of the numerators by the product of the denominators to provide the numerical value for the wanted quantity.

$$\frac{9 \text{ mL}}{\text{hr}} \left| \frac{250 \text{ mg}}{50 \text{ mL}} \right| \frac{1000 \text{ mcg}}{1 \text{ mg}} \left| \frac{1 \text{ hr}}{60 \text{ min}} \right| \frac{2.2 \text{ lb}}{1 \text{ kg}} \left| \frac{}{165 \text{ lb}} \right. = \frac{\text{mcg}}{\text{kg/min}}$$

$$\frac{9 \times 25 \times 100 \times 2.2}{5 \times 6 \times 1 \times 165} \left| \frac{49500}{4950} \right. = \frac{10 \text{ mcg}}{\text{kg/min}}$$

The nurse can inform the physician that the patient is now receiving 10 mcg/kg/min infusing at 9 mL/hr.

> **Practice Exercise 6.1** Involving Dosage, Weight, and Time

1. Order: levothyroxine 10 mcg/kg per dose by mouth every 24 hours to rule out congenital hypothyroidism.
   Supply: levothyroxine 25 mcg/tablet
   Weight of the child: 1.3 kg
   How many tablets per dose will you give? _____

2. Order: Imuran 3 mg/kg/day in three divided doses to prevent renal transplant rejection.
   Supply: Imuran 50 mg/tablet
   Weight of the patient: 210 lb
   How many tablets per dose will you give? _____

3. Information obtained by the nurse: aminophylline 250 mg/250 mL D5W is infusing at 30 mL/hr for a patient weighing 132 lb. How many milligrams per kilogram per hour is the patient receiving? _____

4. Information obtained by the nurse: dopamine 200 mg/250 mL D5W is infusing at 30 mL/hr for a patient weighing 70 kg. How many micrograms per kilogram per minute is the patient receiving? _____

5. Order: milrinone 0.5 mcg/kg/min for short-term treatment of congestive heart failure unresponsive to conventional therapy.
   Supply: milrinone diluted for a concentration 100 mcg/mL in 200 mL of D5W
   Weight of the patient: 80 kg
   Calculate the number of milliliters per hour to set the IV pump. _____

(continued)

Practice Exercise 6.1 Involving Dosage, Weight,
and Time (Continued)

6. Order: dopamine 10 mcg/kg/min to produce car-
   diac stimulation and renal vasodilation.
   Supply: dopamine 200 mg in 500 mL D5W
   Weight of the patient: 110 lb
   Calculate the number of milliliters per hour to set
   the IV pump. _____

7. Order: amrinone 6 mcg/kg/min to increase cardiac
   output.
   Supply: amrinone 100 mg in 100 mL 0.9% NS
   Weight of the patient: 80 kg
   Calculate the number of milliliters per hour to set
   the IV pump. _____

8. Order: esmolol 50 mcg/kg/min for management of
   sinus tachycardia.
   Supply: esmolol 5 g in 500 mL D5W/0.9% NS
   Weight of the patient: 90 kg
   Calculate the number of milliliters per hour to set
   the IV pump. _____

9. Order: nitroprusside 3 mcg/kg/min for manage-
   ment of hypertensive crisis.
   Supply: nitroprusside 200 mg 1000 mL D5W
   Weight of the patient: 70 kg
   Calculate the number of milliliters per hour to set
   the IV pump. _____

10. Order: dobutamine 7.5 mcg/kg/min for short-term
    management of heart failure.
    Supply: dobutamine 1000 mg/1000 mL D5W/0.45
    NaCl
    Weight of the patient: 165 lb
    Calculate the number of milliliters per hour to set
    the IV pump. _____

Solving Problems with Dimensional Analysis

- Dimensional analysis is a problem-solving method that uses critical thinking. When implementing the sequential method or the random method of dimensional analysis, the medication problem can be set up in a number of different ways with a focus on the correct placement of conversion factors to allow unwanted units to be canceled from the unit path.

- Dimensional analysis is a problem-solving method that nurses can use to calculate a variety of medication problems in the hospital, outpatient, or the home-care environment. The medication problems may involve one-factor–, two-factor–, or three-factor–given quantity medication orders resulting in one-factor–, two-factor–, or three-factor–wanted quantity answers.

- With advanced nursing and home-care nursing resulting in increased autonomy, it is more important than ever for nurses to be able to accurately calculate medication problems. Dimensional analysis provides the opportunity to use one problem-solving method for any type of medication problem, thereby increasing consistency and decreasing confusion when calculating medication problems.

SUMMARY

Chapter 6 has helped you to calculate **three-factor** medication problems involving the dosage of medication, the weight of the patient, and the amount of time over which medications or intravenous fluids can be safely administered using the sequential method or the random method of dimensional analysis.

7

PRACTICING PROBLEMS WITH DIMENSIONAL ANALYSIS

This chapter will help you to practice calculating one-factor, two-factor, and three-factor medication problems using dimensional analysis. The goal of this chapter is to clarify that you have a clear understanding of dimensional analysis as a problem-solving method and are capable of solving a variety of medication problems accurately.

ONE-FACTOR PRACTICE PROBLEMS

1. Order: Avandia 8 mg PO daily for control of blood glucose in type 2 diabetes mellitus.
   Supply: Avandia 4 mg tablets
   How many tablets will you give? _____
2. Order: atorvastatin (Lipitor) 20 mg PO daily for management of primary hypercholesterolemia.
   Supply: atorvastatin (Lipitor) 40 mg tablets
   How many tablets will you give? _____
3. Order: lisinopril 5 mg PO daily for management of hypertension.
   Supply: lisinopril 2.5 mg tablets
   How many tablets will you give? _____
4. Order: ketorolac (Toradol) 30 mg IV BID for 24 hours for management of moderately severe acute pain that requires analgesia at the opioid level.
   Supply: ketorolac (Toradol) 15 mg/mL Tubex sterile cartridge
   How many mL will you give? _____
5. Order: ondansetron (Zofran) 4 mg IV every 6 hours for nausea associated with chemotherapy.
   Supply: ondansetron (Zofran) 2 mg/mL vial
   How many mL will you give? _____

6. Order: epoetin (Epogen) 440 units SQ three times weekly for anemia secondary to chronic renal failure.
   Supply: epoetin (Epogen) 2000 units/mL vial
   How many mL will you give? _____

7. Order: cyanocobalamin (vitamin B_{12}) 200 mcg every month for pernicious anemia.
   Supply: cyanocobalamin 100 mcg/mL in 30-mL vials
   How many mL will you give? _____

8. Order: phytonadione (Aquamephyton) 5 mg SC every 12 to 48 hours for treatment of hypoprothrombinemia.
   Supply: phytonadione (Aquamephyton) 10 mg/mL in 1-mL ampules
   How many mL will you give? _____

9. Order: famotidine (Pepcid) 20 mg IV BID for dyspepsia
   Supply: famotidine (Pepcid) 10 mg/mL vial
   How many mL will you give? _____

10. Order: torsemide (Demadex) 10 mg IV daily for management of edema associated with congestive heart failure.
    Supply: torsemide (Demadex) 10 mg/mL in 2 mL ampule
    How many mL will you give? _____

TWO-FACTOR PRACTICE PROBLEMS

1. Order: caffeine citrate 20 mg/kg IV over 30 minutes for apnea of prematurity.
   Supply: caffeine citrate 60 mg/3 mL vial
   Weight of infant: 1.315 kg
   How many mL will you draw from the vial? _____

2. Order: ampicillin 25 mg/kg IV push every 8 hours for respiratory infection secondary to bronchopulmonary dysplasia.
   Supply: ampicillin 1-g vial
   Weight of infant: 3.21 kg

Nursing Drug Reference: Dilute each 1 g with 7.4 mL of sterile water.

How many mL will you draw from the vial after reconstitution? _____

3. Order: heparin 5000 units/hr IV for atrial fibrillation.
   Supply: heparin 25,000 units in 250 mL of NS
   Calculate mL/hr to set the IV pump. _____

4. Order: 1000 mL Lactated Ringers to infuse over 12 hours.
   Supply: 1000 mL Lactated Ringers
   Drop factor: 20 gtt/mL
   Calculate drops per minute (gtt/min). _____

5. Order: 250 mL NS to infuse over 15 minutes.
   Supply: 250 mL NS
   Calculate mL/hr to set the IV pump. _____

6. Order: 1000 mL D5/0.45% NS to infuse over 24 hours.
   Supply: 1000 mL D5/0.45% NS
   Drop factor: 60 gtt/mL
   Calculate drops per minute (gtt/min). _____

7. Information obtained by the nurse: A loading dose of theophylline 1 g/250 mL NS is infusing at 80 mL/hr for a patient weighing 150 lb.
   How many mg/hr is the patient receiving? _____

8. Information obtained by the nurse: 1000 mL D5W/0.9% NS is infusing at 50 gtt/min. The drop factor is 15 gtt/mL. How many hours will it take for the IV to infuse? _____

9. Order: vancomycin 20 mg/kg IV every 12 hours for systemic infection.
   Weight of child: 35 lb
   Supply: vancomycin 500-mg vials
   Nursing drug reference: Dilute each 500-mg vial with 10 mL of sterile water for injection. Further dilute in 100 mL 0.9% NaCl and infuse over 60 minutes.
   How many mL will you draw from the vial after reconstitution? _____
   Calculate mL/hour to set the IV pump. _____

10. Information obtained by the nurse: 150 mg/100 mL
    of amiodarone (Cordarone) is infusing at 600 mL/hr
    for management of life-threatening ventricular
    arrhythmia.

    How many mg/min is the patient receiving? _____

THREE-FACTOR PRACTICE PROBLEMS

1. Order: carbamazepine (Tegretol) 10 mg/kg/day PO
   in 3 divided doses for management of seizures.
   Supply: carbamazepine (Tegretol) 100 mg/5 mL
   Weight of child: 30 kg
   How many mL per dose will you give? _____

2. Order: propranolol (Inderal) 1 mg/kg/day PO in 2
   divided doses for treatment of arrhythmias second-
   ary to heart defect.
   Supply: propranolol (Inderal) 4 mg/mL
   Weight of infant: 2.22 kg
   How many mL per dose will you give? _____

3. Order: gentamicin 4 mg/kg/dose IV every 24 hours
   for gram-negative infection.
   Supply: gentamicin 40 mg/50 mL premixed injec-
   tion slowly over 2 hours
   Weight of infant: 2320 g
   How many mL per dose will you give? _____

4. Information obtained by the nurse: An infant is receiving 60 mg/dose IV every 8 hours of ampicillin.
   Weight of infant: 1200 g
   Nursing drug reference: Recommended dose of ampicillin for neonates under 2 kg is 25–50 mg/kg for
   the first week of life, then 50 mg/kg every 8 hours.
   How many mg/kg/dose is the infant receiving?
   _____

5. Information obtained by the nurse: An infant is receiving 8 mcg/day PO of levothyroxine.
   Weight of infant: 1.315 kg

Nursing drug reference: Recommended dose of levothyroxine for infants under 6 months is 5–6 mcg/day.

How many mcg/kg/day is the infant receiving?

_____

6. Order: aminophylline 0.6 mg/kg/20 min IV loading dose for status asthmaticus followed by 0.36 mg/kg/hr maintenance infusion rate.
   Supply: aminophylline 250 mg in 250 mL NS
   Weight of patient: 95 kg
   How many mL/hour will you set the IV pump for the loading dose? _____
   How many mL/hour will you set the IV pump for the maintenance infusion rate? _____

7. Order: alteplase (Activase) 0.75 mg/kg/30 min IV loading dose for myocardial infarction, followed by 0.5 mg/kg over the next 60 minutes maintenance infusion rate.
   Supply: alteplase (Activase) 100 mg/100 mL
   Weight of patient: 70 kg
   How many mL/hour will you set the IV pump for the loading dose? _____
   How many mL/hour will you set the IV pump for the maintenance infusion rate? _____

8. Information obtained by the nurse: 5 g/500 mL of esmolol (Brevibloc) is infusing at 72 mL/hr for management of supraventricular arrhythmias for a patient weighing 80 kg.
   How many mcg/kg/min is the patient receiving?

_____

9. Order: amrinone (Inocor) 6 mcg/kg/min IV for short-term management of congestive heart failure.
   Supply: amrinone (Inocor) 100 mg/100 mL of 0.9% NaCl
   Weight of the patient: 50 kg
   How many mL/hr will you set the IV pump?

_____

10. Order: nitroprusside (Nipride) 2 mcg/kg/min IV for management of hypertensive crisis.
    Supply: nitroprusside (Nipride) 50 mg/500 mL D5W
    Weight of patient: 220 lb
    How many mL/hour will you set the IV pump?

    _____

SUMMARY

This chapter has provided you with the opportunity for extensive practice with a variety of medication problems using dimensional analysis as a problem-solving method. This chapter also has provided you the opportunity to review one-factor, two-factor, and three-factor medication problems to evaluate your comprehension.

ANSWER KEY FOR PRACTICE EXERCISES

Answers for Chapter 1

Practice Exercise 1.1

1.	$1 + 1$	=	2
2.	$1 - 5$	=	4
3.	$5 + 1$	=	6
4.	10	=	10
5.	$5 + 1 + 1 + 1$	=	8
6.	$10 - 1 + 10$	=	19
7.	$10 + 10$	=	20
8.	$10 + 5 + 1 + 1 + 1$	=	18
9.	1	=	1
10.	$10 + 5$	=	15
11.	$1 + 1 + 1$	=	3
12.	5	=	5
13.	$1 - 10$	=	9
14.	$5 + 1 + 1$	=	7
15.	$10 + 1$	=	11
16.	$10 + 1 - 5$	=	14
17.	$10 + 5 + 1$	=	16
18.	$10 + 1 + 1$	=	12
19.	$10 + 5 + 1 + 1$	=	17
20.	$10 + 1 + 1 + 1$	=	13

Practice Exercise 1.2

1.	34	=	XXXIV
2.	XXII	=	22
3.	75	=	LXXV
4.	XC	=	90
5.	29	=	XXIX
6.	XLII	=	42
7.	56	=	LVI

8. LXIV   =   64
9. 88   =   LXXXVIII
10. CXXI   =   121

Practice Exercise 1.3

1. $\dfrac{3}{4} \times \dfrac{5}{8} = \dfrac{3 \times 5 = 15}{4 \times 8 = 32} = \dfrac{15}{32}$

2. $\dfrac{1}{3} \times \dfrac{4}{9} = \dfrac{1 \times 4 = 4}{3 \times 9 = 27} = \dfrac{4}{27}$

3. $\dfrac{2}{3} \times \dfrac{4}{5} = \dfrac{2 \times 4 = 8}{3 \times 5 = 15} = \dfrac{8}{15}$

4. $\dfrac{3}{4} \times \dfrac{1}{2} = \dfrac{3 \times 1 = 3}{4 \times 2 = 8} = \dfrac{3}{8}$

5. $\dfrac{1}{8} \times \dfrac{4}{5} = \dfrac{1 \times 4 = 4\,(4) = 1}{8 \times 5 = 40\,(4) = 10} = \dfrac{1}{10}$

6. $\dfrac{2}{3} \times \dfrac{5}{8} = \dfrac{2 \times 5 = 10\,(2) = 5}{3 \times 8 = 24\,(2) = 12} = \dfrac{5}{12}$

7. $\dfrac{3}{8} \times \dfrac{2}{3} = \dfrac{3 \times 2 = 6\,(6) = 1}{8 \times 3 = 24\,(6) = 4} = \dfrac{1}{4}$

8. $\dfrac{4}{7} \times \dfrac{2}{4} = \dfrac{4 \times 2 = 8\,(4) = 2}{7 \times 4 = 28\,(4) = 7} = \dfrac{2}{7}$

9. $\dfrac{4}{5} \times \dfrac{1}{2} = \dfrac{4 \times 1 = 4\,(2) = 2}{5 \times 2 = 10\,(2) = 5} = \dfrac{2}{5}$

10. $\dfrac{1}{4} \times \dfrac{1}{8} = \dfrac{1 \times 1 = 1}{4 \times 8 = 32} = \dfrac{1}{32}$

Practice Exercise 1.4

1. $\dfrac{3}{4} \div \dfrac{2}{3} = \dfrac{3}{4} \times \dfrac{3}{2}$ **or** $\dfrac{3 \times 3 = 9}{4 \times 2 = 8} = 1\dfrac{1}{8}$

2. $\dfrac{1}{9} \div \dfrac{3}{9} = \dfrac{1}{9} \times \dfrac{9}{3}$ **or** $\dfrac{1 \times 9 = \ \ 9\,(9) = 1}{9 \times 3 = 27\,(9) = 3} = \dfrac{1}{3}$

3. $\dfrac{2}{3} \div \dfrac{1}{6} = \dfrac{2}{3} \times \dfrac{6}{1}$ **or** $\dfrac{2 \times 6 = 12}{3 \times 1 = 3} = 4$

4. $\dfrac{1}{5} \div \dfrac{4}{5} = \dfrac{1}{5} \times \dfrac{5}{4}$ **or** $\dfrac{1 \times 5 = \ \ 5\,(5) = 1}{5 \times 4 = 20\,(5) = 4} = \dfrac{1}{4}$

5. $\dfrac{3}{6} \div \dfrac{4}{8} = \dfrac{3}{6} \times \dfrac{8}{4}$ **or** $\dfrac{3 \times 8 = 24}{6 \times 4 = 24} = 1$

6. $\dfrac{5}{8} \div \dfrac{5}{8} = \dfrac{5}{8} \times \dfrac{8}{5}$ **or** $\dfrac{5 \times 8 = 40}{8 \times 5 = 40} = 1$

7. $\dfrac{1}{8} \div \dfrac{2}{3} = \dfrac{1}{8} \times \dfrac{3}{2}$ **or** $\dfrac{1 \times 3 = \ 3}{8 \times 2 = 16} = \dfrac{3}{16}$

8. $\dfrac{1}{5} \div \dfrac{1}{2} = \dfrac{1}{5} \times \dfrac{2}{1}$ **or** $\dfrac{1 \times 2 = 2}{5 \times 1 = 5} = \dfrac{2}{5}$

Practice Exercise 1.5

1. 0.75 = 0.8
2. 0.88 = 0.9
3. 0.44 = 0.4
4. 0.23 = 0.2
5. 0.67 = 0.7
6. 0.27 = 0.3
7. 0.98 = 1.0
8. 0.92 = 0.9

Practice Exercise 1.8

1.   2.5   (1 decimal point)
    × _4.6_   (1 decimal point)
       150
      1000
      1150

      11.50   (2 decimal points from the right to left)

2.   1.45   (2 decimal points)
    × _0.25_   (2 decimal points)
       725
      2900
      0000
      3625

      0.3625 (4 decimal points from the right to left)

3.   3.9   (1 decimal point)
    × _0.8_   (1 decimal point)
       312
       000
       312

       3.12   (2 decimal points from the right to left)

4.   2.56   (2 decimal points)
    × _0.45_   (2 decimal points)
       1280
      10240
      00000
      11520

      1.1520 (4 decimal points from the right to left)

5.   10.65   (2 decimal points)
    × _0.05_   (2 decimal points)
       5325
       0000
       5325

       0.5325 (4 decimal points from the right to left)

6.   1.98   (2 decimal points)
 × 3.10   (2 decimal points)
     000
    1980
   59400
   61380

6.1380 (4 decimal points from the right to left)

Practice Exercise 1.7

1. $3.4\overline{)9.6}$

   (Move decimal points one place to the right)

```
     2.82  = 2.8
34.)96.
     68
    280
    272
     80
     68
     12
```

2. $0.25\overline{)12.50}$

   (Move decimal points two places to the right)

```
     50.  = 50
25.)1250.
    125
      0
      0
```

3. $0.56\overline{)18.65}$

   (Move decimal points two places to the right)

$$\begin{array}{r} 33.30 = 33.3 \\ 56.\overline{)1865.} \\ \underline{1680} \\ 185 \\ \underline{168} \\ 170 \\ \underline{168} \\ 20 \end{array}$$

4. $0.3\overline{)0.192}$

   (Move decimal points one place to the right)

$$\begin{array}{r} .64 = 0.6 \\ 3.\overline{)01.92} \\ \underline{18} \\ 12 \\ \underline{12} \end{array}$$

5. $0.4\overline{)12.43}$

   (Move decimal points one place to the right)

$$\begin{array}{r} 31.075 = 31.1 \\ 4.\overline{)124.3} \\ \underline{12} \\ 4 \\ \underline{4} \\ 3 \\ \underline{0} \\ 30 \\ \underline{28} \\ 20 \\ \underline{20} \end{array}$$

6. $0.5\overline{)12.50}$

(Move decimal points one place to the right)

$$5.\overline{)125.0}$$
$$\begin{array}{r} 25 \\ \hline 125.0 \\ \underline{10} \\ 25 \\ \underline{25} \end{array}$$

7. $0.125\overline{)0.25}$

(Move decimal points three places to the right)

$$125.\overline{)250.} = 2$$
$$\begin{array}{r} 2 \\ \hline 250. \\ \underline{250} \end{array}$$

8. $0.08\overline{)0.085}$

(Move decimal points two places to the right)

$$8.\overline{)8.5} = 1.1$$
$$\begin{array}{r} 1.0625 \\ \hline 8.5 \\ \underline{8} \\ 5 \\ \underline{0} \\ 50 \\ \underline{48} \\ 20 \\ \underline{16} \\ 40 \\ \underline{40} \end{array}$$

Practice Exercise 1.8

1. $\dfrac{1}{8}$ = $8\overline{)1.0}$ = 0.125

$$
\begin{array}{r}
0.125 \\
8\overline{)1.0} \\
\underline{8} \\
20 \\
\underline{16} \\
40 \\
\underline{40}
\end{array}
$$

2. $\dfrac{1}{4}$ = $4\overline{)1.0}$ = 0.25

$$
\begin{array}{r}
0.25 \\
4\overline{)1.0} \\
\underline{8} \\
20 \\
\underline{20}
\end{array}
$$

3. $\dfrac{2}{5}$ = $5\overline{)2.0}$ = 0.4

$$
\begin{array}{r}
0.4 \\
5\overline{)2.0} \\
\underline{20}
\end{array}
$$

4. $\dfrac{3}{5}$ = $5\overline{)3.0}$ = 0.6

$$
\begin{array}{r}
0.6 \\
5\overline{)3.0} \\
\underline{30}
\end{array}
$$

5. $\dfrac{2}{3}$ = $3\overline{)2.0}$ = 0.66

$$
\begin{array}{r}
0.66 \\
3\overline{)2.0} \\
\underline{18} \\
20 \\
\underline{18} \\
2
\end{array}
$$

6. $\dfrac{6}{8} = 8\overline{)6.00}^{\,0.75} = 0.75$

$$\begin{array}{r} \underline{56} \\ 40 \\ \underline{40} \end{array}$$

7. $\dfrac{3}{8} = 8\overline{)3.00}^{\,0.375} = 0.375$

$$\begin{array}{r} \underline{24} \\ 60 \\ \underline{56} \\ 40 \\ \underline{40} \end{array}$$

8. $\dfrac{1}{3} = 3\overline{)1.00}^{\,0.33} = 0.33$

$$\begin{array}{r} \underline{9} \\ 10 \\ \underline{9} \\ 1 \end{array}$$

9. $\dfrac{3}{6} = 6\overline{)3.0}^{\,0.5} = 0.5$

$$\underline{30}$$

10. $\dfrac{2}{10} = 10\overline{)2.0}^{\,0.2} = 0.2$

$$\underline{20}$$

Answers for Chapter 2

Practice Exercise 2.1

1. kilogram	=	kg
2. gram	=	g
3. milligram	=	mg
4. microgram	=	mcg
5. liter	=	L
6. milliliter	=	mL
7. cubic centimeter	=	cc

Practice Exercise 2.2

1. pound	=	lb
2. ounce	=	oz
3. dram	=	dr
4. grain	=	gr
5. gallon	=	gal
6. quart	=	qt
7. pint	=	pt
8. fluid ounce	=	fl oz
9. fluid dram	=	fl dr
10. minim	=	M

Practice Exercise 2.3

1. tablespoon	=	tbsp
2. teaspoon	=	tsp
3. drop	=	gtt

Practice Exercise 2.4

1. 1 kg	=	2.2 lb		
2. 1 kg	=	1000 g		
3. 1 g	=	1000 mg		
4. 1 mg	=	1000 mcg		
5. 1 g	=	15 gr		
6. 1 gr	=	60 mg		
7. 1000 mg	=	1 g		
8. 1000 mL	=	1 L	=	1 qt

9. 500 mL   =   1 pt
10. 240 mL   =   8 oz
11. 30 mL   =   1 oz   =   2 tbsp
12. 15 mL   =   ½ oz   =   3 tsp
13. 5 mL   =   1 tsp
14 1 mL   =   15 M   =   15 gtt
15. 1 mL   =   1 cc

Answers for Chapter 3

Practice Exercise 3.1

1. Problem: 4 mg   =   How many g?
   Given quantity   =   4 mg
   Wanted quantity   =   g
   Conversion factor   =   1 g = 1000 mg

$$\frac{4 \text{ mg}}{} \left| \frac{1 \text{ g}}{1000 \text{ mg}} \right| \frac{4 \times 1}{1000} \right| \frac{4}{1000} = 0.004 \text{ g}$$

2. Problem: 5000 g   =   How many kg?
   Given quantity   =   5000 g
   Wanted quantity   =   kg
   Conversion factor   =   1 kg = 1000 g

$$\frac{5000 \text{ g}}{} \left| \frac{1 \text{ kg}}{1000 \text{ g}} \right| \frac{5 \times 1}{1} \right| \frac{5}{1} = 5 \text{ kg}$$

3. Problem: 0.3 L   =   How many cc?
   Given quantity   =   0.3 L
   Wanted quantity   =   cc
   Conversion factor   =   1 L = 1000 cc

$$\frac{0.3 \text{ L}}{} \left| \frac{1000 \text{ cc}}{1 \text{ L}} \right| \frac{0.3 \times 1000}{1} \right| \frac{300}{1} = 300 \text{ cc}$$

4. Problem: 10 cc   =   How many mL?
   Given quantity   =   10 cc
   Wanted quantity   =   mL
   Conversion factor   =   1 cc = 1 mL

$$\frac{10 \text{ cc} \quad | \quad 1 \text{ mL}}{\quad | \quad 1 \text{ cc}} \quad \frac{10 \times 1}{1} \quad \frac{10}{1} = 10 \text{ mL}$$

5. Problem: 120 lb   =   How many kg?
   Given quantity   =   120 lb
   Wanted quantity   =   kg
   Conversion factor   =   2.2 lb = 1 kg

$$\frac{120 \text{ lb} \quad | \quad 1 \text{ kg}}{\quad | \quad 2.2 \text{ lb}} \quad \frac{120 \times 1}{2.2} \quad \frac{120}{2.2} = 54.5 \text{ kg}$$

6. Problem: 5 gr   =   How many mg?
   Given quantity   =   5 gr
   Wanted quantity   =   mg
   Conversion factor   =   1 gr = 60 mg

$$\frac{5 \text{ gr} \quad | \quad 60 \text{ mg}}{\quad | \quad 1 \text{ gr}} \quad \frac{5 \times 60}{1} \quad \frac{300}{1} = 300 \text{ mg}$$

7. Problem: 2 g   =   How many gr?
   Given quantity   =   2 g
   Wanted quantity   =   gr
   Conversion factor   =   1 g = 15 gr

$$\frac{2 \text{ g} \quad | \quad 15 \text{ gr}}{\quad | \quad 1 \text{ g}} \quad \frac{2 \times 15}{1} \quad \frac{30}{1} = 30 \text{ gr}$$

8. Problem: 5 fl dr   =   How many mL?
   Given quantity   =   5 fl dr
   Wanted quantity   =   mL
   Conversion factor   =   1 fl dr = 5 mL

$$\frac{5 \text{ fl dr} \quad | \quad 5 \text{ mL}}{\quad | \quad 1 \text{ fl dr}} \quad \frac{5 \times 5}{1} \quad \frac{25}{1} = 25 \text{ mL}$$

9. Problem: 8 fl dr   =   How many fl oz?
   Given quantity   =   8 fl dr
   Wanted quantity   =   fl oz
   Conversion factor   =   1 fl dr = 5 mL
   Conversion factor   =   1 fl oz = 30 mL

$$\frac{8\ \text{fl dr}}{} \left| \frac{5\ \text{mL}}{1\ \text{fl dr}} \right| \frac{1\ \text{(fl oz)}}{30\ \text{mL}} \right| \frac{8 \times 5 \times 1}{1 \times 30} \right| \frac{40}{30} = 1.3\ \text{fl oz}$$

10. Problem: 10 M   =   How many fl dr?
    Given quantity   =   M
    Wanted quantity   =   fl dr
    Conversion factor   =   1 mL = 15 M
    Conversion factor   =   1 fl dr = 5 mL

$$\frac{10\ \text{M}}{} \left| \frac{1\ \text{mL}}{15\ \text{M}} \right| \frac{1\ \text{(fl dr)}}{5\ \text{mL}} \right| \frac{10 \times 1 \times 1}{15 \times 5} \right| \frac{10}{75} = 0.13\ \text{fl dr}$$

11. Problem: 35 kg   =   How many lb?
    Given quantity   =   35 kg
    Wanted quantity   =   lb
    Conversion factor   =   1 kg = 2.2 lb

$$\frac{35\ \text{kg}}{} \left| \frac{2.2\ \text{(lb)}}{1\ \text{kg}} \right| \frac{35 \times 2.2}{1} \right| \frac{77}{1} = 77\ \text{lb}$$

12. Problem: 10 mL   =   How many tsp?
    Given quantity   =   10 mL
    Wanted quantity   =   tsp
    Conversion factor   =   1 tsp = 5 mL

$$\frac{10\ \text{mL}}{} \left| \frac{1\ \text{(tsp)}}{5\ \text{mL}} \right| \frac{10 \times 1}{5} \right| \frac{10}{5} = 2\ \text{tsp}$$

13. Problem: 30 mL   =   How many tbsp?
    Given quantity   =   30 mL
    Wanted quantity   =   tbsp
    Conversion factor   =   1 tbsp = 15 mL

$$\frac{30\ \text{mL}}{} \left| \frac{1\ \text{(tbsp)}}{15\ \text{mL}} \right| \frac{30 \times 1}{15} \right| \frac{30}{15} = 2\ \text{tbsp}$$

14. Problem: 0.25 g   =   How many mg?
    Given quantity   =   0.25 g
    Wanted quantity   =   mg
    Conversion factor   =   1 g = 1000 mg

$$\frac{0.25 \text{ g}}{} \; \bigg| \; \frac{1000 \text{ (mg)}}{1 \text{ g}} \; \bigg| \; \frac{0.25 \times 1000}{1} \; \bigg| \; \frac{250}{1} = 250 \text{ mg}$$

15. Problem: 350 mcg   =   How many mg?
    Given quantity   =   350 mcg
    Wanted quantity   =   mg
    Conversion factor   =   1 mg = 1000 mcg

$$\frac{350 \text{ mcg}}{} \; \bigg| \; \frac{1 \text{ (mg)}}{1000 \text{ mcg}} \; \bigg| \; \frac{350 \times 1}{1000} \; \bigg| \; \frac{350}{1000} = 0.35 \text{ mg}$$

16. Problem: 0.75 L   =   How many mL?
    Given quantity   =   0.75 L
    Wanted quantity   =   mL
    Conversion factor   =   1 L = 1000 mL

$$\frac{0.75 \text{ L}}{} \; \bigg| \; \frac{1000 \text{ (mL)}}{1 \text{ L}} \; \bigg| \; \frac{0.75 \times 1000}{1} \; \bigg| \; \frac{750}{1} = 750 \text{ mL}$$

17. Problem: 3 hr   =   How many min?
    Given quantity   =   3 hr
    Wanted quantity   =   min
    Conversion factor   =   1 hr = 60 min

$$\frac{3 \text{ hr}}{} \; \bigg| \; \frac{60 \text{ (min)}}{1 \text{ hr}} \; \bigg| \; \frac{3 \times 60}{1} \; \bigg| \; \frac{180}{1} = 180 \text{ min}$$

18. Problem: 3.5 mL   =   How many M?
    Given quantity   =   3.5 mL
    Wanted quantity   =   M
    Conversion factor   =   1 mL = 15 M

$$\frac{3.5 \text{ mL}}{} \; \bigg| \; \frac{15 \text{ (M)}}{1 \text{ mL}} \; \bigg| \; \frac{3.5 \times 15}{1} \; \bigg| \; \frac{52.5}{1} = 52.5 \text{ M}$$

19. Problem: 500 mcg   =   How many mg?
    Given quantity   =   500 mcg
    Wanted quantity   =   mg
    Conversion factor   =   1 mg = 1000 mcg

$$\frac{500 \text{ mcg}}{} \left| \frac{1 \text{ (mg)}}{1000 \text{ mcg}} \right| \frac{500 \times 1}{1000} \left| \frac{500}{1000} \right. = 0.5 \text{ mg}$$

20. Problem: 225 M   =   How many tsp?
    Given quantity   =   225 M
    Wanted quantity   =   tsp
    Conversion factor =   1 mL = 15 M
    Conversion factor =   1 tsp = 5 mL

$$\frac{225 \text{ M}}{} \left| \frac{1 \text{ mL}}{15 \text{ M}} \right| \frac{1 \text{ (tsp)}}{5 \text{ mL}} \left| \frac{225 \times 1 \times 1}{15 \times 5} \right| \frac{225}{75} = 3 \text{ tsp}$$

Answers for Chapter 4

Practice Exercise 4.1

Medication Order #1

1. Right **patient**   Mr. S. Smith
2. Right **drug**   Advil (ibuprofen) for arthritis
3. Right **dosage**   400 mg
4. Right **route**   PO (orally)
5. Right **time**   every 6 hrs

Medication Order #2

1. Right **patient**   Mr. J. Jones
2. Right **drug**   Tylenol (acetaminophen)
                         for headache
3. Right **dosage**   gr 10
4. Right **route**   PO (orally)
5. Right **time**   every 4 hrs/PRN

Practice Exercise 4.2

Sequential method

1. $\dfrac{7.5 \text{ mg}}{} \left| \dfrac{\text{(tablet)}}{5 \text{ mg}} \right| \dfrac{7.5}{5} = 1.5$ tablets

Sequential method

2. $\dfrac{100 \text{ mg}}{} \cdot \left| \dfrac{\text{(tablet)}}{50 \text{ mg}} \right| \dfrac{10}{5} = 2$ tablets

Random method

3. $\dfrac{0.075 \text{ mg}}{} \left| \dfrac{\text{(tablet)}}{75 \text{ mcg}} \right| \dfrac{1000 \text{ mcg}}{1 \text{ mg}} \left| \dfrac{0.075 \times 1000}{75 \times 1} \right| \dfrac{75}{75}$

= 1 tablet

Sequential method

4. $\dfrac{8 \text{ mg}}{} \left| \dfrac{\text{(tablet)}}{4 \text{ mg}} \right| \dfrac{8}{4} = 2$ tablets

Sequential method

5. $\dfrac{40 \text{ mg}}{} \left| \dfrac{\text{(tablet)}}{80 \text{ mg}} \right| \dfrac{4}{8} = \frac{1}{2}$ tablet

Practice Exercise 4.3

Augmentin

a. Trade name of the drug: Augmentin
b. Generic name of the drug: amoxicillin/clavulanate potassium tablets
c. Dosage of medication: 250 mg
d. Form of medication: tablets
e. Expiration date: Abbreviation display (number not listed)
f. Lot or batch number: Abbreviation display (number not listed)
g. Manufacturer: SmithKline Beecham Pharmaceuticals

Zaroxolyn

a. Trade name of the drug: Zaroxolyn
b. Generic name of the drug: metolazone
c. Dosage of medication: 10 mg
d. Form of medication: tablets
e. Expiration date: Abbreviation display
                                    (number not listed)
f. Lot or batch number: Abbreviation display
                                    (number not listed)
g. Manufacturer: Fisons Pharmaceuticals

Practice Exercise 4.4

Random method

1. $\dfrac{0.25 \text{ mg}}{} \bigg| \dfrac{\text{tablet}}{125 \text{ mcg}} \bigg| \dfrac{1000 \text{ mcg}}{1 \text{ mg}} \bigg| \dfrac{0.25 \times 1000}{125 \times 1} \bigg| \dfrac{250}{125}$

   = 2 tablets

Sequential method

2. $\dfrac{500 \text{ mg}}{} \bigg| \dfrac{\text{tablet}}{250 \text{ mg}} \bigg| \dfrac{50}{25} = 2 \text{ tablets}$

Sequential method

3. $\dfrac{2.5 \text{ mg}}{} \bigg| \dfrac{\text{tablet}}{5 \text{ mg}} \bigg| \dfrac{2.5}{5} = \frac{1}{2} \text{ tablet}$

Sequential method

4. $\dfrac{150 \text{ mg}}{} \bigg| \dfrac{\text{tablet}}{150 \text{ mg}} \bigg| \dfrac{15}{15} = 1 \text{ tablet}$

Sequential method

5. $\dfrac{30 \text{ mg}}{} \bigg| \dfrac{\text{tablet}}{15 \text{ mg}} \bigg| \dfrac{30}{15} = 2 \text{ tablets}$

Practice Exercise 4.5

Sequential method

1. $\dfrac{30\ mg}{} \left| \dfrac{5\ \text{(mL)}}{20\ mg} \right| \dfrac{3 \times 5}{2} \left| \dfrac{15}{2} \right. = 7.5$ mL

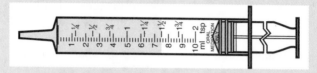

Sequential method

2. $\dfrac{325\ mg}{} \left| \dfrac{20.3\ \text{(mL)}}{650\ mg} \right| \dfrac{325 \times 20.3}{650} \left| \dfrac{6597.5}{650} \right. = 10.15$ or 10 mL

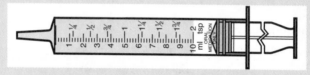

Sequential method

3. $\dfrac{30\ g}{} \left| \dfrac{30\ \text{(mL)}}{20\ g} \right| \dfrac{3 \times 30}{2} \left| \dfrac{90}{2} \right. = 45$ mL

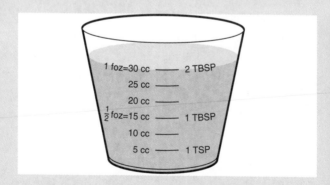

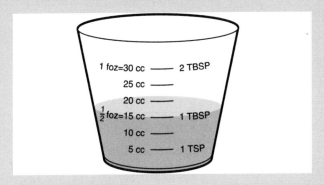

Sequential method

4. $\dfrac{15\ \text{mL}}{} \left| \dfrac{1\ \text{tsp}}{5\ \text{mL}} \right| \dfrac{15 \times 1}{5} \quad \dfrac{15}{5} = 3\ \text{tsp}$

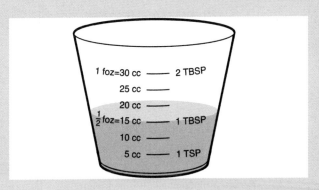

Random method

5. $\dfrac{0.05\ \text{mg}}{} \left| \dfrac{\text{mL}}{50\ \text{mcg}} \right| \dfrac{1000\ \text{mcg}}{1\ \text{mg}} \left| \dfrac{0.05 \times 100}{5 \times 1} \right| \dfrac{5}{5} = 1\ \text{mL}$

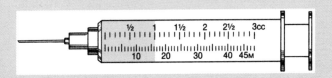

Practice Exercise 4.6

Sequential method

1. $\dfrac{300 \text{ mg}}{} \quad \Big| \quad \dfrac{2 \text{(mL)}}{300 \text{ mg}} \quad \Big| \quad \dfrac{2}{} \quad = 2 \text{ mL}$

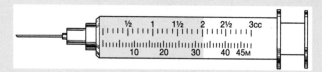

Random method

2. $\dfrac{1000 \text{ mg}}{} \quad \Big| \quad \dfrac{2 \text{(mL)}}{1 \text{ g}} \quad \Big| \quad \dfrac{1 \text{ g}}{1000 \text{ mg}} \quad \Big| \quad \dfrac{2}{} \quad = 2 \text{ mL}$

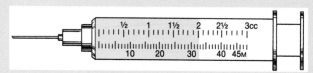

Sequential method

3. $\dfrac{200 \text{ mg}}{} \quad \Big| \quad \dfrac{\text{(mL)}}{100 \text{ mg}} \quad \Big| \quad \dfrac{2}{1} \quad = 2 \text{ mL}$

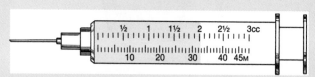

Sequential method

4. $\dfrac{10 \text{(units)}}{} \quad \Big| \quad 10 \qquad\qquad = 10 \text{ units}$

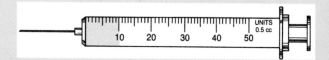

Sequential method

5. $\dfrac{5000 \text{ units}}{} \left| \dfrac{\text{(mL)}}{10,000 \text{ units}} \right| \dfrac{5}{10} = 0.5 \text{ mL}$

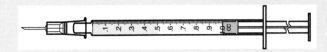

Answers for Chapter 5

Practice Exercise 5.1

Sequential method

1. $\dfrac{15 \text{ mg}}{\text{kg}} \left| \dfrac{\text{(tablet)}}{250 \text{ mg}} \right| \dfrac{1 \text{ kg}}{2.2 \text{ lb}} \left| 85 \text{ lb} \right| \dfrac{15 \times 1 \times 85}{250 \times 2.2} \left| \dfrac{1275}{550} \right.$

= 2.318 or 2 tablets

Sequential method

2. $\dfrac{0.3 \text{ mg}}{\text{kg}} \left| \dfrac{10 \text{ (mL)}}{20 \text{ mg}} \right| 40 \text{ kg} \left| \dfrac{0.3 \times 10 \times 4}{2} \right| \dfrac{12}{2} = 6 \text{ mL}$

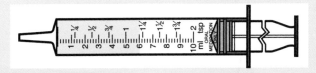

Sequential method

3. $\dfrac{100 \text{ units}}{\text{kg}} \left| \dfrac{\text{(mL)}}{10,000 \text{ units}} \right| \dfrac{1 \text{ kg}}{2.2 \text{ lb}} \left| 100 \text{ lb} \right| \dfrac{10 \times 1 \times 1}{10 \times 2.2} \left| \dfrac{10}{22} \right.$

= 0.45 or 0.5 mL

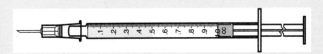

Sequential method

4. $\dfrac{1 \text{ mg}}{\text{kg}} \quad \left| \dfrac{\text{mL}}{10 \text{ mg}} \quad \right| \dfrac{20 \text{ kg}}{} \quad \left| \dfrac{1 \times 2}{1} = 2 \text{ mL}\right.$

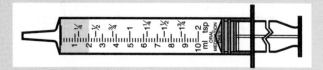

Sequential method

5. $\dfrac{6 \text{ mcg}}{\text{kg}} \quad \left| \dfrac{\text{mL}}{300 \text{ mcg}} \quad \right| \dfrac{50 \text{ kg}}{} \quad \left| \dfrac{6 \times 5}{30} \quad \right| \dfrac{30}{30} = 1 \text{ mL}\right.$

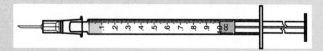

Practice Exercise 5.2

Sequential method

1. $\dfrac{600 \text{ mg}}{} \quad \left| \dfrac{5 \text{ mL}}{100 \text{ mg}} \quad \right| \dfrac{6 \times 5}{1} \quad \left| \dfrac{30}{1} = 30 \text{ mL}\right.$

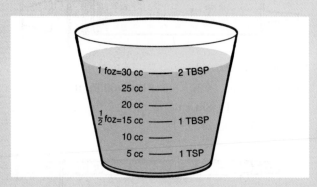

Sequential method

2. $\dfrac{12.5 \text{ mg}}{\text{kg}} \left| \dfrac{5 \text{ (mL)}}{125 \text{ mg}} \right| \dfrac{1 \text{ kg}}{2.2 \text{ lb}} \left| 22 \text{ lb} \right| \dfrac{12.5 \times 5 \times 1 \times 22}{125 \times 2.2} \dfrac{1375}{275}$

= 5 mL

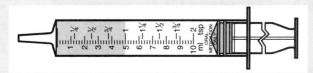

Sequential method

3. $\dfrac{33.3 \text{ mg}}{\text{kg}} \left| \dfrac{1 \text{ kg}}{2.2 \text{ lb}} \right| 50 \text{ lb} \left| \dfrac{10 \text{ (mL)}}{500 \text{ mg}} \right| \dfrac{33.3 \times 1 \times 5 \times 1}{2.2 \times 5} \dfrac{166.5}{11}$

= 15.13 or 15 mL

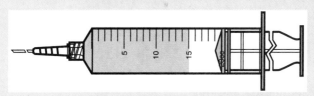

Sequential method

4. $\dfrac{50 \text{ mg}}{\text{kg}} \left| \dfrac{5 \text{ (mL)}}{500 \text{ mg}} \right| 25 \text{ kg} \left| \dfrac{5 \times 5 \times 25}{50} \dfrac{625}{50} \right| = 12.5$ mL

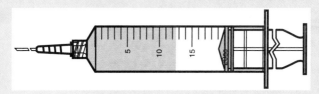

Sequential method

$$5. \quad \frac{7.5 \text{ mg}}{\text{kg}} \begin{vmatrix} 75 \text{ kg} \end{vmatrix} \frac{10 \text{ (mL)}}{500 \text{ mg}} \begin{vmatrix} \frac{7.5 \times 75 \times 1}{50} \end{vmatrix} \frac{562.5}{50} = \frac{11.25 \text{ or}}{11 \text{ mL}}$$

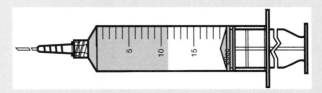

Sequential method

$$1. \quad \frac{2500 \text{ units}}{\text{(hr)}} \begin{vmatrix} \frac{250 \text{ (mL)}}{25,000 \text{ units}} \end{vmatrix} \frac{25}{} = \frac{25 \text{ mL}}{\text{hr}}$$

Random method

$$2. \quad \frac{54 \text{ mg}}{\text{(hr)}} \begin{vmatrix} 250 \text{ (mL)} \\ 1 \text{ g} \end{vmatrix} \frac{1 \text{ g}}{1000 \text{ mg}} \begin{vmatrix} \frac{54 \times 25 \times 1}{1 \times 100} \end{vmatrix} \frac{1350}{100} = \frac{13.5 \text{ mL}}{\text{hr}}$$

Sequential method

$$3. \quad \frac{22 \text{ units}}{\text{(hr)}} \begin{vmatrix} \frac{100 \text{ (mL)}}{100 \text{ units}} \end{vmatrix} \frac{22}{} = \frac{22 \text{ mL}}{\text{hr}}$$

Sequential method

$$4. \quad \frac{10 \text{ mg}}{\text{(hr)}} \begin{vmatrix} \frac{\text{(mL)}}{1 \text{ mg}} \end{vmatrix} \frac{10}{1} = \frac{10 \text{ mL}}{\text{hr}}$$

Sequential method

$$5. \quad \frac{20 \text{ mg}}{\text{(hr)}} \begin{vmatrix} \frac{\text{(mL)}}{2 \text{ mg}} \end{vmatrix} \frac{20}{2} = \frac{10 \text{ mL}}{\text{hr}}$$

Practice Exercise 5.4

Sequential method

1.

1000 mL	1 hr	20 gtt	$1000 \times 1 \times 2$	2000
12 hr	60 min	mL	12×6	72

$$= 27.7 \text{ or } 28 \frac{\text{gtt}}{\text{min}}$$

Sequential method

2.

250 mL	10 gtt	250×1	250	
30 min	mL	3	3	$= 83.3 \text{ or } 83 \frac{\text{gtt}}{\text{min}}$

Sequential method

3.

1000 mL	20 gtt	min	1 hr	$10 \times 20 \times 1$	200
	mL	50 gtt	60 min	5×6	30

$$= 6.66 \text{ or } 6 \text{ hr}$$

Sequential method

4.

500 mL	10 gtt	1 hr	$500 \times 1 \times 1$	500
8 hr	mL	60 min	8×6	48

$$= 10.41 \text{ or } 10 \frac{\text{gtt}}{\text{min}}$$

Sequential method

5.

150 mL	20 gtt	1 hr	$150 \times 2 \times 1$	300	
hr	mL	60 min	6	6	$= 50 \frac{\text{gtt}}{\text{min}}$

Practice Exercise 5.5

Random method

1.

500 mg	10 mL	1 g	$5 \times 1 \times 1$	5	
	1 g	1000 mg	1×1	1	$= 5 \text{ mL}$

Sequential method

105 mL	60 min	105	$= 105 \dfrac{\text{mL}}{\text{hr}}$
60 min	1 hr	1	

Sequential method

$$\frac{105 \text{ mL}}{\text{hr}} \left| \frac{20 \text{ gtt}}{\text{mL}} \right| \frac{1 \text{ hr}}{60 \text{ min}} \left| \frac{105 \times 2 \times 1}{6} \right| \frac{210}{6} = \frac{35 \text{ gtt}}{\text{min}}$$

Sequential method

$$2.\ \frac{1 \text{ g}}{} \left| \frac{10 \text{ mL}}{1 \text{ g}} \right| \frac{10}{} = 10 \text{ mL}$$

Sequential method

$$\frac{110 \text{ mL}}{60 \text{ min}} \left| \frac{60 \text{ min}}{1 \text{ hr}} \right| \frac{110}{1} = \frac{110 \text{ mL}}{\text{hr}}$$

Sequential method

$$\frac{110 \text{ mL}}{\text{hr}} \left| \frac{20 \text{ gtt}}{\text{mL}} \right| \frac{1 \text{ hr}}{60 \text{ min}} \left| \frac{110 \times 2 \times 1}{6} \right| \frac{220}{6} = 36.66 \text{ or } 37 \frac{\text{gtt}}{\text{min}}$$

Random method

$$3.\ \frac{500 \text{ mg}}{} \left| \frac{10 \text{ mL}}{1 \text{ g}} \right| \frac{1 \text{ g}}{1000 \text{ mg}} \left| \frac{5}{1} = 5 \text{ mL} \right.$$

Sequential method

$$\frac{205 \text{ mL}}{60 \text{ min}} \left| \frac{60 \text{ min}}{1 \text{ hr}} \right| \frac{205}{1} = \frac{205 \text{ mL}}{\text{hr}}$$

Sequential method

$$\frac{205 \text{ mL}}{\text{hr}} \left| \frac{20 \text{ gtt}}{\text{mL}} \right| \frac{1 \text{ hr}}{60 \text{ min}} \left| \frac{205 \times 2 \times 1}{6} \right| \frac{410}{6} = 68.33 \text{ or } 68 \frac{\text{gtt}}{\text{min}}$$

Sequential method

$$4.\ \frac{300 \text{ mg}}{} \left| \frac{4 \text{ mL}}{600 \text{ mg}} \right| \frac{3 \times 4}{6} \left| \frac{12}{6} = 2 \text{ mL} \right.$$

Sequential method

$$\frac{52 \text{ mL}}{20 \text{ min}} \left| \frac{60 \text{ min}}{1 \text{ hr}} \right| \frac{52 \times 6}{2 \times 1} \left| \frac{312}{2} = 156 \frac{\text{mL}}{\text{hr}} \right.$$

Sequential method

$$\frac{156 \text{ mL}}{\text{hr}} \left| \frac{20 \text{ (gtt)}}{\text{mL}} \right| \frac{1 \text{ hr}}{60 \text{ (min)}} \left| \frac{156 \times 2 \times 1}{6} \right| \frac{312}{6} = \frac{52 \text{ gtt}}{\text{min}}$$

Sequential method

$$5. \frac{3 \text{ g}}{} \left| \frac{10 \text{ (mL)}}{3 \text{ g}} \right| \frac{10}{} = 10 \text{ mL}$$

Sequential method

$$\frac{110 \text{ (mL)}}{30 \text{ min}} \left| \frac{60 \text{ min}}{1 \text{ (hr)}} \right| \frac{110 \times 6}{3 \times 1} \left| \frac{660}{3} \right| = \frac{220 \text{ mL}}{\text{hr}}$$

Sequential method

$$\frac{220 \text{ mL}}{\text{hr}} \left| \frac{20 \text{ (gtt)}}{\text{mL}} \right| \frac{1 \text{ hr}}{60 \text{ (min)}} \left| \frac{220 \times 2 \times 1}{6} \right| \frac{440}{6} = 73.33 \text{ or } 73 \frac{\text{gtt}}{\text{min}}$$

Answers for Chapter 6

Practice Exercise 6.1

Sequential method

$$1. \frac{10 \text{ mcg}}{\text{kg/(dose)}} \left| \frac{1.3 \text{ kg}}{} \right| \frac{\text{(tablet)}}{25 \text{ mcg}} \left| \frac{10 \times 1.3}{25} \right| \frac{13}{25}$$

$$= \frac{0.52 \text{ or } \frac{1}{2} \text{ tablet}}{\text{dose}}$$

Sequential method

$$2. \frac{3 \text{ mg}}{\text{kg/day}} \left| \frac{\text{(tablet)}}{50 \text{ mg}} \right| \frac{1 \text{ kg}}{2.2 \text{ lb}} \left| \frac{210 \text{ lb}}{} \right| \frac{\text{day}}{3 \text{ (dose)}} \left| \frac{1 \times 210}{50 \times 2.2} \right| \frac{210}{110}$$

$$= \frac{1.9 \text{ or } 2 \text{ tablets}}{\text{dose}}$$

Sequential method

3. 30 mL	250 mg		2.2 lb	30 × 2.2	66
hr	250 mL	132 lb	1 kg	132 × 1	132

$$= \frac{0.5 \text{ mg}}{\text{kg/hr}}$$

Sequential method

4. 30 mL	200 mg	1 hr	1000 mcg		30 × 20 × 10
hr	250 mL	60 min	1 mg	70 kg	25 × 6 × 7

$$\frac{6000}{1050} = 5.7 \frac{\text{mcg}}{\text{kg/min}}$$

Sequential method

5. 0.5 mcg	mL	80 kg	60 min	0.5 × 8 × 6	24
kg/min	100 mcg		1 hr	1 × 1	1

$$= \frac{24 \text{ mL}}{\text{hr}}$$

Random method

6. 10 mcg	1 kg	110 lb	1 mg	500 mL	60 min
kg/min	2.2 lb		1000 mcg	200 mg	1 hr

$$\frac{1 \times 11 \times 5 \times 6}{2.2 \times 2} \quad \frac{330}{44} = 7.5 \frac{\text{mL}}{\text{hr}}$$

Sequential method

7. 6 mcg	80 kg	60 min	100 mL	1 mg	6 × 8 × 6
kg/min		1 hr	100 mg	1000 mcg	10

$$\frac{288}{10} = 28.8 \frac{\text{mL}}{\text{hr}}$$

Sequential method

8. $\dfrac{50 \text{ mcg}}{\text{kg/min}} \left| \dfrac{90 \text{ kg}}{} \right| \dfrac{60 \text{ min}}{1\,\text{hr}} \left| \dfrac{1 \text{ mg}}{1000 \text{ mcg}} \right| \dfrac{500\,\text{mL}}{5\,\text{g}} \left| \dfrac{1\,\text{g}}{1000\,\text{mg}} \right.$

$\dfrac{5 \times 9 \times 6 \times 5}{5 \times 10} \left| \dfrac{1350}{50} = 27 \dfrac{\text{mL}}{\text{hr}} \right.$

Sequential method

9. $\dfrac{3 \text{ mcg}}{\text{kg/min}} \left| \dfrac{70 \text{ kg}}{} \right| \dfrac{60 \text{ min}}{1\,\text{hr}} \left| \dfrac{1 \text{ mg}}{1000 \text{ mcg}} \right| \dfrac{1000\,\text{mL}}{200 \text{ mg}} \left| \dfrac{3 \times 7 \times 6}{2} \right.$

$\dfrac{126}{2} = 63 \dfrac{\text{mL}}{\text{hr}}$

10. $\dfrac{7.5 \text{ mcg}}{\text{kg/min}} \left| \dfrac{60 \text{ min}}{1\,\text{hr}} \right| \dfrac{1\,\text{kg}}{2.2\,\text{lb}} \left| \dfrac{165\,\text{lb}}{} \right| \dfrac{1 \text{ mg}}{1000 \text{ mcg}} \left| \dfrac{1000\,\text{mL}}{1000\,\text{mg}} \right.$

$\dfrac{7.5 \times 6 \times 1 \times 165}{2.2 \times 100} \left| \dfrac{7425}{220} = 33.75 \text{ or } 33.8 \dfrac{\text{mL}}{\text{hr}} \right.$

Answers for Chapter 7

One-Factor Practice Problems

1. $\dfrac{8 \text{ mg}}{} \left| \dfrac{\text{tablet}}{4 \text{ mg}} \right| \dfrac{8}{4} = 2 \text{ tablets}$

2. $\dfrac{20 \text{ mg}}{} \left| \dfrac{\text{tablet}}{40 \text{ mg}} \right| \dfrac{2}{4} = 0.5 \text{ or } \tfrac{1}{2} \text{ tablet}$

3. $\dfrac{5 \text{ mg}}{} \left| \dfrac{\text{tablet}}{2.5 \text{ mg}} \right| \dfrac{5}{2.5} = 2 \text{ tablets}$

4. $\dfrac{30 \text{ mg}}{} \left| \dfrac{\text{mL}}{15 \text{ mg}} \right| \dfrac{30}{15} = 2 \text{ mL}$

5. $\dfrac{4 \text{ mg}}{} \left| \dfrac{\text{mL}}{2 \text{ mg}} \right| \dfrac{4}{2} = 2 \text{ mL}$

6. $\dfrac{440 \text{ units}}{} \left|\dfrac{\text{(mL)}}{2000 \text{ units}}\right| \dfrac{44}{200} = 0.22$ or 0.2 mL

7. $\dfrac{200 \text{ mcg}}{} \left|\dfrac{\text{(mL)}}{100 \text{ mcg}}\right| \dfrac{2}{1} = 2$ mL

8. $\dfrac{5 \text{ mg}}{} \left|\dfrac{\text{(mL)}}{10 \text{ mg}}\right| \dfrac{5}{10} = 0.5$ mL

9. $\dfrac{20 \text{ mg}}{} \left|\dfrac{\text{(mL)}}{10 \text{ mg}}\right| \dfrac{2}{1} = 2$ mL

10. $\dfrac{10 \text{ mg}}{} \left|\dfrac{\text{(mL)}}{10 \text{ mg}}\right| \dfrac{1}{1} = 1$ mL

Two-Factor Practice Problems

1. $\dfrac{20 \text{ mg}}{\text{kg}} \left|\dfrac{3 \text{(mL)}}{60 \text{ mg}}\right| 1.315 \text{ kg} \left|\dfrac{2 \times 3 \times 1.315}{6}\right| \dfrac{7.89}{6} = \dfrac{1.315 \text{ or}}{1.3 \text{ mL}}$

2. $\dfrac{25 \text{ mg}}{\text{kg}} \left|\dfrac{7.4 \text{(mL)}}{1 \text{ g}}\right| 3.21 \text{ kg} \left|\dfrac{1 \text{ g}}{1000 \text{ mg}}\right| \dfrac{25 \times 7.4 \times 3.21}{1000}$

$\dfrac{593.85}{1000} = 0.59385$ or 0.6 mL

3. $\dfrac{5000 \text{ units}}{\text{(hr)}} \left|\dfrac{250 \text{(mL)}}{25,000 \text{ units}}\right| \dfrac{50}{} = \dfrac{50 \text{ mL}}{\text{hr}}$

4. $\dfrac{1000 \text{ mL}}{12 \text{ hr}} \left|\dfrac{20 \text{(gtt)}}{\text{mL}}\right| \dfrac{1 \text{ hr}}{60 \text{(min)}} \dfrac{1000 \times 2 \times 1}{12 \times 6} \dfrac{2000}{72}$

$= \dfrac{27.77 \text{ or } 28 \text{ gtt}}{\text{min}}$

5. $\dfrac{250 \text{(mL)}}{15 \text{ min}} \left|\dfrac{60 \text{ min}}{1 \text{(hr)}}\right| \dfrac{250 \times 60}{15 \times 1} \dfrac{15,000}{15} = \dfrac{1000 \text{ mL}}{\text{hr}}$

6. $\dfrac{1000 \text{ mL}}{24 \text{ hr}} \bigg| \dfrac{60 \text{ (gtt)}}{\text{mL}} \bigg| \dfrac{1 \text{ hr}}{60 \text{ (min)}} \bigg| \dfrac{1000 \times 1}{24} \bigg| \dfrac{1000}{24}$

$= \dfrac{41.666 \text{ or } 42 \text{ gtt}}{\text{min}}$

7. $\dfrac{80 \text{ mL}}{\text{(hr)}} \bigg| \dfrac{1 \text{ g}}{250 \text{ mL}} \bigg| \dfrac{1000 \text{ (mg)}}{1 \text{ g}} \bigg| \dfrac{80 \times 100}{25} \bigg| \dfrac{8000}{25} = 320 \dfrac{\text{mg}}{\text{hr}}$

8. $\dfrac{1000 \text{ mL}}{} \bigg| \dfrac{15 \text{ gtt}}{\text{mL}} \bigg| \dfrac{\text{min}}{50 \text{ gtt}} \bigg| \dfrac{1 \text{ (hr)}}{60 \text{ min}} \bigg| \dfrac{10 \times 15 \times 1}{5 \times 6} \bigg| \dfrac{150}{30} = 5 \text{ hr}$

9. $\dfrac{20 \text{ mg}}{\text{kg}} \bigg| \dfrac{10 \text{ (mL)}}{500 \text{ mg}} \bigg| \dfrac{35 \text{ lb}}{} \bigg| \dfrac{1 \text{ kg}}{2.2 \text{ lb}} \bigg| \dfrac{2 \times 1 \times 35 \times 1}{5 \times 2.2} \bigg| \dfrac{70}{11}$

$= 6.36 \text{ or } 6.4 \text{ mL}$

10. $\dfrac{106.4 \text{ (mL)}}{60 \text{ min}} \bigg| \dfrac{60 \text{ min}}{1 \text{ (hr)}} = \dfrac{106.4 \text{ mL}}{\text{hr}}$

$\dfrac{600 \text{ mL}}{\text{hr}} \bigg| \dfrac{150 \text{ (mg)}}{100 \text{ mL}} \bigg| \dfrac{1 \text{ hr}}{60 \text{ (min)}} \bigg| \dfrac{6 \times 15 \times 1}{1 \times 6} \bigg| \dfrac{90}{6} = 15 \dfrac{\text{mg}}{\text{min}}$

Three-Factor Practice Problems

1. $\dfrac{10 \text{ mg}}{\text{kg/day}} \bigg| \dfrac{5 \text{ (mL)}}{100 \text{ mg}} \bigg| \dfrac{30 \text{ kg}}{} \bigg| \dfrac{\text{day}}{3 \text{ (doses)}} \bigg| \dfrac{5}{} = 5 \dfrac{\text{mL}}{\text{dose}}$

2. $\dfrac{1 \text{ mg}}{\text{kg/day}} \bigg| \dfrac{\text{(mL)}}{4 \text{ mg}} \bigg| \dfrac{2.22 \text{ kg}}{} \bigg| \dfrac{\text{day}}{2 \text{ (doses)}} \bigg| \dfrac{1 \times 2.22}{4 \times 2} \bigg| \dfrac{2.22}{8}$

$= \dfrac{0.2775 \text{ or } 0.3 \text{ mL}}{\text{dose}}$

3. $\dfrac{4 \text{ mg}}{\text{kg/(dose)}} \bigg| \dfrac{50 \text{ (mL)}}{40 \text{ mg}} \bigg| \dfrac{1 \text{ kg}}{1000 \text{ g}} \bigg| \dfrac{2320 \text{ g}}{} \bigg| \dfrac{4 \times 5 \times 1 \times 232}{40 \times 10} \bigg| \dfrac{4640}{400}$

$= \dfrac{11.6 \text{ mL}}{\text{dose}}$

4. $\dfrac{60 \text{ (mg)}}{\text{(dose)}} \bigg| \dfrac{1000 \text{ g}}{1 \text{ (kg)}} \bigg| \dfrac{}{1200 \text{ g}} \bigg| \dfrac{60 \times 10}{1 \times 12} \bigg| \dfrac{600}{12} = 50 \dfrac{\text{mg}}{\text{kg/dose}}$

5. $\dfrac{8\,\boxed{\text{mcg}}}{\boxed{\text{day}}} \Bigg| \dfrac{}{1.315\,\boxed{\text{kg}}} \Bigg| \dfrac{8}{1.315} = 6.08 \text{ or } 6 \dfrac{\text{mcg}}{\text{kg/day}}$

6. $\dfrac{0.6\,\text{mg}}{\text{kg/20 min}} \Bigg| \dfrac{250\,\boxed{\text{mL}}}{250\,\text{mg}} \Bigg| \dfrac{95\,\text{kg}}{} \Bigg| \dfrac{60\,\text{min}}{1\,\boxed{\text{hr}}} \Bigg| \dfrac{0.6 \times 95 \times 6}{2 \times 1} \Bigg| \dfrac{342}{2}$

$= 171 \dfrac{\text{mL}}{\text{hr}}$

$\dfrac{0.36\,\text{mg}}{\text{kg/hr}} \Bigg| \dfrac{250\,\boxed{\text{mL}}}{250\,\text{mg}} \Bigg| \dfrac{95\,\text{kg}}{} \Bigg| \dfrac{0.36 \times 95}{} = 34.2 \dfrac{\text{mL}}{\text{hr}}$

7. $\dfrac{0.75\,\text{mg}}{\text{kg/30 min}} \Bigg| \dfrac{100\,\boxed{\text{mL}}}{100\,\text{mg}} \Bigg| \dfrac{70\,\text{kg}}{} \Bigg| \dfrac{60\,\text{min}}{1\,\boxed{\text{hr}}} \Bigg| \dfrac{0.75 \times 70 \times 6}{3 \times 1} \Bigg| \dfrac{315}{3}$

$= 105 \dfrac{\text{mL}}{\text{hr}}$

$\dfrac{0.5\,\text{mg}}{\text{kg/60 min}} \Bigg| \dfrac{100\,\boxed{\text{mL}}}{100\,\text{mg}} \Bigg| \dfrac{70\,\text{kg}}{} \Bigg| \dfrac{60\,\text{min}}{1\,\boxed{\text{hr}}} \Bigg| \dfrac{0.5 \times 70}{1} = 35 \dfrac{\text{mL}}{\text{hr}}$

8. $\dfrac{72\,\text{mL}}{\text{hr}} \Bigg| \dfrac{5\,\text{g}}{500\,\text{mL}} \Bigg| \dfrac{1\,\text{hr}}{60\,\boxed{\text{min}}} \Bigg| \dfrac{1000\,\text{mg}}{1\,\text{g}} \Bigg| \dfrac{1000\,\boxed{\text{mcg}}}{1\,\text{mg}} \Bigg| \dfrac{}{80\,\boxed{\text{kg}}}$

$\dfrac{72 \times 5 \times 10 \times 10}{5 \times 6 \times 1 \times 8} \Bigg| \dfrac{36,000}{240} = 150 \dfrac{\text{mcg}}{\text{kg/min}}$

9. $\dfrac{6\,\text{mcg}}{\text{kg/min}} \Bigg| \dfrac{100\,\boxed{\text{mL}}}{100\,\text{mg}} \Bigg| \dfrac{1\,\text{mg}}{1000\,\text{mcg}} \Bigg| \dfrac{50\,\text{kg}}{} \Bigg| \dfrac{60\,\text{min}}{1\,\boxed{\text{hr}}} \Bigg| \dfrac{6 \times 5 \times 6}{10}$

$\dfrac{180}{10} = 18 \dfrac{\text{mL}}{\text{hr}}$

10. $\dfrac{2\,\text{mcg}}{\text{kg/min}} \Bigg| \dfrac{500\,\boxed{\text{mL}}}{50\,\text{mg}} \Bigg| \dfrac{1\,\text{mg}}{1000\,\text{mcg}} \Bigg| \dfrac{1\,\text{kg}}{2.2\,\text{lb}} \Bigg| \dfrac{220\,\text{lb}}{} \Bigg| \dfrac{60\,\text{min}}{1\,\boxed{\text{hr}}}$

$\dfrac{2 \times 22 \times 6}{2.2} \Bigg| \dfrac{264}{2.2} = 120 \dfrac{\text{mL}}{\text{hr}}$

Abbreviations Used in Clinical Calculations

ā *or* a	before
ac	before meals
ad lib	as desired, freely
AM	in the morning, before noon
bid	twice a day
c̄	with
cap *or* caps	capsule
cc	cubic centimeter
cm	centimeter
dr *or* ℥	dram
DC	discontinue
DX	diagnosis
D5W	dextrose 5% in water
D5/$\frac{1}{2}$NS	dextrose 5% in water with 0.45% normal saline
elix	elixir
et	and
fl *or* fld	fluid
g *or* gm	gram
gal	gallon
gr	grain
gtt	drop
h *or* hr	hour
hs	hour of sleep (bedtime)
IM	intramuscular(ly)
inj	injection
iss	$1\frac{1}{2}$ or one and a half
IV	intravenous(ly)
IVPB	intravenous piggyback
kg	kilogram
KCl	potassium chloride
KVO	keep vein open
L	liter
lb	pound
liq	liquid
m	meter
M *or* M̨	minim
mcg	microgram
mEq	milliequivalent

mg	milligram
min	minute
mL	milliliter
NPO	nothing by mouth
NS	normal saline, sodium chloride or 0.9% NS
OD	right eye
OS	left eye
os	mouth
oz *or* $\overline{z}_3$	ounce
OU	both eyes
$\bar{p}$	after
p	per
PB	piggyback
pc	after meals
per	by
po *or* per os	by mouth
PM	afternoon or evening
prn	as needed or when necessary
pt	pint
q	every
qd	every day
qh	every hour
q2h	every 2 hours
q3h	every 3 hours
q4h	every 4 hours
q6h	every 6 hours
q8h	every 8 hours
qid	four times a day
qod	every other day
qt	quart
R	rectal
R/O	rule out
RX	treatment
$\bar{s}$	without
SC	subcutaneous(ly)
SL	sublingual (beneath the tongue)
SQ	subcutaneous(ly)
ss	$\frac{1}{2}$ or half
stat	immediately or at once
supp	suppository
tab	tablet
tbs, tbsp, T	tablespoon
tid	three times a day
TKO	to keep open
tsp, t	teaspoon
U	unit

Guidelines for Selecting Needles

NEEDLE GAUGE AND LENGTHS	USAGE
23 to 25 gauge	Thin liquid medications
21 to 22 gauge	Thick liquid medications
$\frac{5}{8}$ to 1 inch	Infants
1 to 1½ inch	Older children
1 to 1½ inch	Adults

Guidelines for Injections

SUBCUTANEOUS INJECTIONS

Syringe and Needle Sizes to Use
- Syringe: 1-3 mL
- Needle gauge: 25-28 gauge
- Needle length: ½ to ⅝ inch

Injection Sites to Use
- Outer aspect of the upper arm
- Abdomen (level with or below the navel)
- Back above the waist
- Anterior thigh

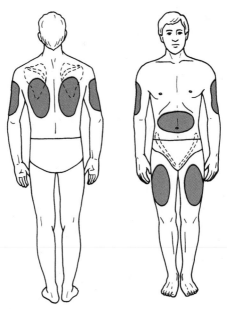

Subcutaneous injection sites.

Subcutaneous Site Rotation Chart

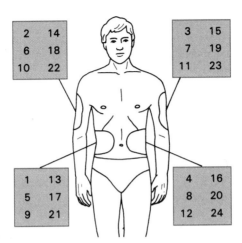

(**A**) Nurse using arm and abdomen. (**B**) Patient using abdomen and thighs.

Procedure to Follow

Wear gloves. Inject into the loose connective tissue underneath the skin; do not inject more than 2 mL at a time. Areas of the body that can be "pinched up" are best suited—abdomen, upper thigh, upper arm. The needle is inserted at 45 degrees or 90 degrees; the plunger is pulled back to ensure that no blood returns and the needle is not in a vein. If no blood returns, inject solution. Subcutaneous sites should be rotated for frequent injections. Monitor sites for signs of abscess or necrotic tissue. Do not use this method for patients in shock, and monitor patients with poor perfusion or low blood pressure, as the drug may not be absorbed or may be absorbed very slowly.

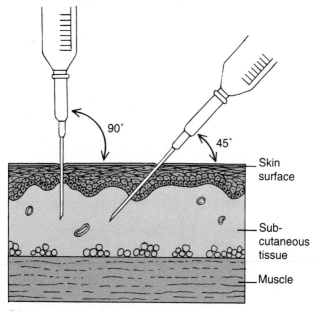

Subcutaneous injection deposits medication in subcutaneous tissue at a 45- or 90-degree angle.

INTRAMUSCULAR INJECTIONS

Syringe and Needle Sizes to Use
- Syringe: 3-5 mL
- Gauges: 20-22 gauge
- Needle length: 1 to 1½ inch

Injection Sites to Use
- Dorsogluteal
- Ventrogluteal
- Vastus lateralis
- Deltoid

Landmarks for Intramuscular Injection Sites

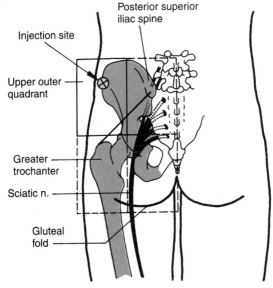

A. Dorsogluteal site.

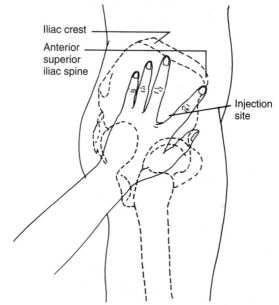

B. Ventrogluteal site.

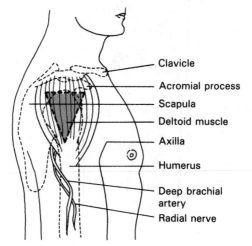

C. Deltoid site.

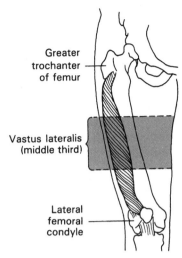

Greater trochanter of femur

Vastus lateralis (middle third)

Lateral femoral condyle

D. Vastus lateralis site.

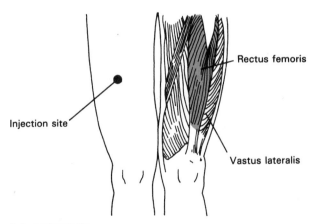

Rectus femoris

Injection site

Vastus lateralis

E. Rectus femoris site.

Procedure to Follow

Wear gloves. Insert needle quickly into big muscle; pull the plunger back to assure that no blood returns and the needle is not in a vein. If no blood returns, inject slowly. Position the patient to relax the muscle, which will increase blood flow, aid absorption, and decrease pain. Vastus lateralis muscle of the thigh is site of choice for children up to 3 yr; ventrogluteal muscle is the site of choice for older children and adults; deltoid muscle and gluteus maximus are other possible sites in special situations.

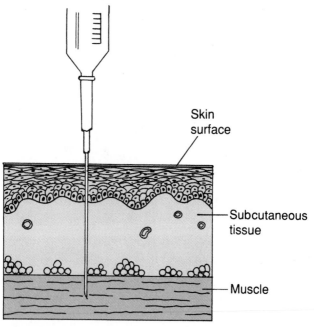

The intramuscular injection deposits medication into the muscle at a 90-degree angle.

INTRADERMAL INJECTIONS

Syringes and Needle Sizes to Use
- Syringe: 1 mL
- Needle gauge: 25-27 gauge
- Needle length: ¼ to ⅝ inch

Injection Sites to Select
- Ventral forearm
- Upper chest
- Upper back below the scapulae

Procedure to Follow
Wear gloves. Inject directly below the surface of the skin. The injection should produce a wheal or fluid-filled bump that can be seen beneath the skin at the injection site. Skin on the back of the forearm is the usual site for these injections. The area should be marked or mapped for reading tests in 24–48 hours.

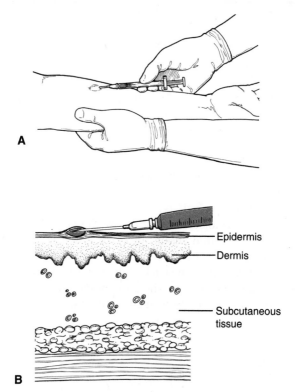

A

B

— Epidermis

— Dermis

— Subcutaneous tissue

(**A**) For intradermal injection, the syringe is held almost parallel to the skin with the bevel up. (**B**) A small volume of medication is deposited right under the skin, forming a small bleb.

Z-TRACK INJECTIONS

Syringe and Needle Sizes to Use
- Syringe: 3-5 mL
- Needle gauge: 19-22 gauge
- Needle length: 1 inch to draw up medication and add 0.5 mL air into the syringe (0.2 mL for infants). Then switch to 2–3 inch.

Injection Site to Use
- Dorsogluteal

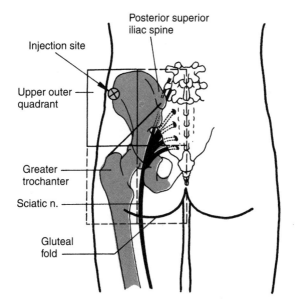

Posterior superior iliac spine

Injection site

Upper outer quadrant

Greater trochanter

Sciatic n.

Gluteal fold

Procedure to Follow

Very irritating or staining solutions may be given by Z-track technique. Wearing gloves, the skin is prepped and pulled very tightly to one side; the needle is inserted into the muscle. The drug is injected as the needle is withdrawn slowly and the skin released. This procedure allows the various overlapping layers of tissue to slide back into position in a Z formation, sealing off the injected material.

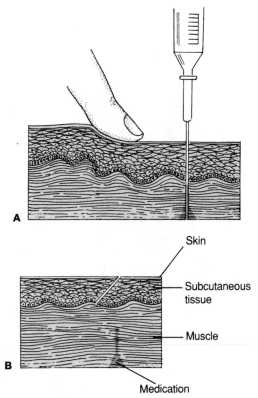

Z-track method. (**A**) Pull skin and subcutaneous tissue 1 to 1.5 inches to side of injection site while injecting medication. (**B**) Release traction to allow skin to fall back, sealing medication in site.

Laboratory Values and Signs and Symptoms of Electrolyte Imbalances

NORMAL LEVEL ADULT VALUES	IMBALANCE	SIGNS AND SYMPTOMS
Na+ 135–145 mEq/L Required in acid-base and osmotic pressure balance, nerve function, and water equilibrium	Decreased	Hypotension, headache, nausea, vomiting, abdominal cramps, muscle tremors, twitching, fatigue, diarrhea, weakness, confusion, seizures, coma
	Increased	Lethargy, irritability, muscle twitching, tremors, dry skin and mucous membranes, fever, hypotension, disorientation, delirium, cerebral hemorrhage, coma
K+ 3.5–5 mEq/L Major factor in carbohydrate metabolism, osmotic pressure balance, acid-base balance and normal muscle contraction	Decreased	Cardiac arrhythmia, depressed S-T segment, flattened/inverted T wave, development of a U wave, confusion, lethargy, muscle weakness, paralysis, abdominal distention, constipation, paralytic ileus, thirst, frequent voiding
	Increased	Muscle weakness, paralysis, numbness and tingling, ventricular fibrillation, cardiac arrest, tall tented T waves
Ca++ 8.5–10 mg/dL Involved in bone and tooth formation, blood coagulation, nerve function, muscle contraction	Decreased	Frequent hives, chronic fatigue, canker and cold sores, muscle cramps (charley horses), itchy skin, dementia, depression, psychosis, tetany (Chvostek's and Trousseau's signs),

NORMAL LEVEL ADULT VALUES	IMBALANCE	SIGNS AND SYMPTOMS
		laryngospasm, generalized convulsions, cardiac arrhythmias with lengthened QT segments
	Increased	Muscle weakness, bone fragility, kidney stones, loss of appetite, thirst, frequent urination, lethargy, fatigue, joint pains, memory loss, depression, constipation, anorexia, nausea and vomiting, abdominal pain, ileus, polyuria, nocturia, polydipsia, emotional lability, confusion, delirium, psychosis, stupor, coma, cardiac arrhythmias with shortened QT segments
Mg^{2+} 1.3–2.1 mEq/L Required for activation of an enzyme necessary for energy metabolism and bone formation	Decreased	Muscle weakness, fatigue, confusion, restlessness, hyperexcitability, vertigo, seizures, muscle tremors, nystagmus, tachycardia, hypotension, premature atrial contraction, premature ventricular contraction, anorexia, nausea, vomiting, personality change, tetany (eg, positive Trousseau's or Chvostek's sign or spontaneous carpopedal spasm), tremor and muscle fasciculations
	Increased	Muscle weakness, drowsiness, lethargy, hypotension, paralysis, coma, cardiac and respiratory problems

Signs and Symptoms of Hypoglycemia and Hyperglycemia

NORMAL LEVEL ADULT VALUES	IMBALANCE	SIGNS AND SYMPTOMS
Blood glucose Fasting blood glucose: 70–100 mg/dL 2-hr postprandial: 90–140 mg/dL Random blood glucose: 70–160 mg/dL	Hypoglycemia	• Restlessness • Irritability • Confusion • Trembling • Slurred speech • Headache • Tingling lips • Paresthesia • Diaphoresis (cool skin) • Pallor • Tachycardia • Shallow respirations • Hypertension • Weakness • Hunger • Coma • Tremors
	Hyperglycemia	• Fatigue • Flushed, dry skin • Dry mouth • Increased thirst • Increased urination • Blurry vision • Headache • Nausea and vomiting • Dehydration • Weak, rapid pulse • Hypotension • High blood glucose levels (>240 mg/dL)
	Diabetic ketoacidosis	• Ketones in urine • Increased thirst and urination • Nausea, vomiting, and/or stomach pain

NORMAL LEVEL ADULT VALUES	IMBALANCE	SIGNS AND SYMPTOMS
		• Changes in or difficulty breathing (Kussmaul's respirations)
		• Acid or fruity smell on breath (acetone breath)
		• Flushing
		• Dehydration
		• Fatigue
		• Stupor and coma

Laboratory Values and Signs and Symptoms of Acid-Base Imbalances

IMBALANCE	CAUSES	SIGNS AND SYMPTOMS	TREATMENT
Respiratory acidosis Caused by excessive accumulation of carbon dioxide, resulting in excessive acidity of body fluids • $<$ pH • $>$ HCO_3 • $>$ $PaCO_2$	Lung disease, including chronic obstructive pulmonary disease	Shortness of breath, fatigue, chronic cough or wheezing, confusion, irritability, or lethargy	Bronchodilators, oxygen, and mechanical ventilation
Respiratory alkalosis Caused by excessive loss of carbon dioxide, resulting in excessive alkalinity of body fluids • $>$ pH • $<$ HCO_3 • $<$ $PaCO_2$	Lung conditions that result from decreased oxygen in the blood, including hyperventilation (anxiety, fever, exercise) and mechanical overventilation	Confusion, muscle twitching, hand tremors, nausea, vomiting, lightheadedness, and paresthesia of the extremities	Breathe into a paper bag to cause retention of carbon dioxide and readjust ventilator settings
Metabolic acidosis Caused by excessive acidity of body fluids • $<$ pH • $<$ HCO_3 • $<$ $PaCO_2$	Kidney failure, poisoning, diabetic ketoacidosis (DKA), starvation, severe diarrhea,	Shortness of breath, lethargy, and confusion	Replace sodium bicarbonate

IMBALANCE	CAUSES	SIGNS AND SYMPTOMS	TREATMENT
	severe dehydration, excessive intake of aspirin, and shock		
Metabolic alkalosis Caused by excessive accumulation of alkaline (bicarbonate) in the blood • > pH • > HCO$_3$ • > PaCO$_2$	Severe vomiting, excessive gastric suctioning, excessive use of antacids, laxatives or steroids, and potassium-wasting diuretics	Cyanosis, nausea, vomiting, irritability, twitching, confusion, tachycardia, hypotension, convulsions, and coma	Replace fluids, potassium; ECG monitoring; drugs to regulate heart rate and blood pressure, drugs to control nausea and vomiting

ARTERIAL BLOOD GAS VALUES

pH	7.35 to 7.45
PaO$_2$ (partial pressure of oxygen)	80 to 100 mm Hg
PaCO$_2$ (partial pressure of carbon dioxide)	35 to 45 mm Hg
SaO$_2$ (oxygen saturation)	97% to 100%
HCO$_3$ (bicarbonate)	22 to 26 mEq/L
Pulse oximetry	95% to 100%

mm Hg, millimeters of mercury; mEq/L, milliequivalents per liter.

Insulin Table: Onset, Peak, and Duration

INSULIN	ONSET	PEAK	DURATION
Regular IV	10–30 min	15–30 min	30–60 min
Regular SQ	30 min–1 hr	2–4 hr	5–7 hr
Intermediate (NPH and Lente)	1–3 hr	6–12 hr	18–28 hr
Long-lasting (Ultralente)	4–6 hr	18–24 hr	36 hr

HYPOGLYCEMIA

Signs and symptoms of hypoglycemia include mental confusion, hallucinations, convulsions, tachycardia, anxiety, and pale, cool, clammy skin.

Monitor patients closely for onset of hypoglycemia reaction during the peak phase following administration of insulin. Mild hypoglycemia can be treated with ingestion of oral glucose. Severe hypoglycemia is life-threatening and is considered a medical emergency. It must be treated with IV glucose, glucagon, or epinephrine.

HYPERGLYCEMIA

Signs and symptoms of hyperglycemia include polyuria, polydipsia, polyphagia, and hot, red, dry skin.

Monitor patients closely for the onset of hyperglycemia. Treatment of mild hyperglycemia includes insulin administration. Severe hyperglycemia may be caused by missing, miscalculating, or mistiming doses of insulin or oral medication, or by overeating or drinking. It is life-threatening and must be treated with administration of SQ or IV insulin and IV fluid replacement.

Blood Administration: Complications With Signs and Symptoms and Treatment

TYPES OF REACTIONS	SIGNS AND SYMPTOMS	TREATMENT
Allergic reaction Most common reaction between the recipient's immune system and foreign plasma proteins in the donated blood	Flushing, pruritus, urticaria	Diphenhydramine (Benadryl) can help reduce the symptoms.
Febrile reaction This type of reaction is caused by antibodies in the recipient's plasma attacking white blood cells in the donated blood or sensitivity to donor WBCs, platelets, or plasma proteins	Sudden chills and fever, headache, flushing, anxiety, muscle pain	Acetaminophen (Tylenol) may help reduce the symptoms. Avoid aspirin in thrombocytopenic patients. Use leukocyte-poor blood products (filtered, washed, or frozen to remove WBCs from the donated blood).
Acute hemolytic reaction Most serious reaction that occurs because of ABO incompatibility between the donor and recipient. The recipient's antibodies attack the transfused RBCs causing them to hemolyze, which in turn releases harmful substances that	Chills, fever, low back pain, flushing, tachycardia, tachypnea, hypotension, vascular collapse, hemoglobinuria, hemoglobinemia, bleeding, acute renal failure, shock, cardiac arrest, death	Obtain blood and urine samples to send to laboratory. Treatment includes monitoring the patient's ECG, BP, cardiac output, and urine output. Maintain volume and blood pressure through infusion of crystalloids. Give diuretics to maintain urine output.

TYPES OF REACTIONS	SIGNS AND SYMPTOMS	TREATMENT
can cause damage to the kidneys		Insert catheter to measure hourly urine output.
Delayed hemolytic reaction This type of reaction occurs when the recipient's antibodies attack antigens (other than ABO antigens) on the transfused blood cells. As the transfused blood cells are destroyed, the patient begins to develop symptoms. This type of reaction can occur days to weeks after the transfusion	Fever, jaundice, anemia, fatigue, and hematuria	Usually no treatment is necessary.
Anaphylactic reaction	Anxiety, urticaria, wheezing, progressing to cyanosis, shock, and cardiac arrest	Initiate CPR. Epinephrine (0.4 mL of a 1:1000 solution SQ or 0.1 mL of 1:1000 solution diluted to 10 mL with saline for IV).
Circulatory overload	Cough, dyspnea, pulmonary congestion, rales, headache, hypertension, tachycardia, and distended neck veins	Position patient upright with feet in dependent position. Administer diuretics, oxygen, and morphine.
Sepsis	Rapid onset of chills, high fever, vomiting, diarrhea, hypotension, and shock	Obtain blood samples to send to laboratory.

Frequently Used Drugs With Corresponding Laboratory Values

DRUG	THERAPEUTIC AND TOXIC LEVELS*
Acetaminophen (Tylenol)	Therapeutic: 1–30 mcg/mL Toxic: >200 mcg/mL
Alcohol (ethanol)	Therapeutic: 100 mcg/mL Toxic: >400 mcg/mL
Aminoglycosides (gentamicin, neomycin, streptomycin, tobramycin, vancomycin)	Trough: 2–10 mcg/mL (varies with drug) Trough levels are referred to as the minimum drug concentration that precedes the administration of a single dose of medication. Trough levels should be drawn just prior to the next dose. Peak: 10–35 mcg/mL (varies with drug) Peak levels are referred to as the maximum drug concentration that follows the administration of a single dose of medication. Peak levels should be drawn 1 hour after IM injections and 30 minutes after a 30-minute IV infusion is completed.
Amitriptyline (Elavil)	Therapeutic: 120–250 mcg/mL Toxic: >500 mcg/mL
Carbamazepine (Tegretol)	Therapeutic: 8–12 mcg/mL Toxic: >15 mcg/mL
Chlordiazepoxide (Librium)	Therapeutic: 700–1000 mcg/mL Toxic: >5000 mcg/mL
Disopyramide (Norpace)	Therapeutic: Variable Toxic: >7 mcg/mL
Diazepam (Valium)	Therapeutic: 100–1000 mcg/mL Toxic: >5000 mcg/mL
Digitoxin	Therapeutic: 20–35 ng/mL Toxic: >45 ng/mL
Digoxin	Therapeutic: 0.8–1.5 mcg/mL Toxic: >2 mcg/mL
Doxepin	Therapeutic: 30–150 mcg/mL Toxic: >500 mcg/mL

DRUG	THERAPEUTIC AND TOXIC LEVELS*
Imipramine (Tofranil)	Therapeutic: 125–250 mcg/mL Toxic: >500 mcg/mL
Lithium	Therapeutic: 0.6–1.2 mcg/mL Toxic: >2 mcg/mL
Lidocaine (Xylocaine)	Therapeutic: 1.5–6 mcg/mL Toxic: >6–8 mcg/mL
Methotrexate	Therapeutic: Variable Toxic: >454 mcg/mL (48 hours after high dose)
Phenobarbital	Therapeutic: 15–40 mcg/mL Toxic: Varies 35–80 mcg/mL
Phenytoin (Dilantin)	Therapeutic: 10–20 mcg/mL Toxic: Varies with symptoms
Procainamide (Pronestyl)	Therapeutic: 5–12 mcg/mL Toxic: >15 mcg/mL
Primidone (Mysoline)	Therapeutic: 5–10 mcg/mL Toxic: >15 mcg/mL
Quinidine	Therapeutic: 2–6 mcg/mL Toxic: >8 mcg/mL
Theophylline	Therapeutic: 10–20 mcg/mL Toxic: >20 mcg/mL
Valproic acid (Depakene)	Therapeutic: 50–100 mcg/mL Toxic: >100 mcg/mL

*Levels vary between laboratories.

DEA Schedules of Controlled Substances

The Controlled Substances Act of 1970 regulates the manufacturing, distribution, and dispensing of drugs that are known to have abuse potential. The Drug Enforcement Agency (DEA) is responsible for the enforcement of these regulations. The controlled drugs are divided into five DEA schedules based on their potential for abuse and physical and psychological dependence.

Schedule I *(C-I):* High abuse potential and no accepted medical use (heroin, marijuana, LSD)

Schedule II *(C-II):* High abuse potential with severe dependence liability (narcotics, amphetamines, and barbiturates)

Schedule III *(C-III):* Less abuse potential than schedule II drugs and moderate dependence liability (nonbarbiturate sedatives, nonamphetamine stimulants, limited amounts of certain narcotics)

Schedule IV *(C-IV):* Less abuse potential than schedule III and limited dependence liability (some sedatives, antianxiety agents, and nonnarcotic analgesics)

Schedule V *(C-V):* Limited abuse potential. Primary small amounts of narcotics (codeine) used as antitussives or antidiarrheals. Under federal law, limited quantities of certain Schedule V drugs may be purchased without a prescription directly from a pharmacist. The purchaser must be at least 18 years of age and must furnish suitable identification. All such transactions must be recorded by the dispensing pharmacist.

Prescribing physicians and dispensing pharmacists must be registered with the DEA, which also provides forms for the transfer of Schedule I and II substances and establishes criteria for the inventory and prescribing of controlled substances. State and local laws are often more stringent than federal law. In any given situation, the more stringent law applies.

Quick Reference Dietary Guidelines

There are specific food sources that the nurse must be knowledgeable about and include in the nutritional teaching for clients.

FOOD TYPE	FOOD SOURCES
Potassium-rich foods	Dried fruits, fresh fruits and juices, garlic, ginger root, whole grains, molasses, potatoes, salad and vegetable produce, flour
Calcium-rich foods	Brown rice, buttermilk, canned salmon, sardines, cheese, figs, almonds, oats, sesame seeds, sunflower seeds, tofu, dairy and soy yogurt
Sodium-rich foods	Bouillon, condiments, canned meats, canned vegetables, canned soups, cured meats, frozen dinners, luncheon meats, pickled vegetables, preseasoned rice and pasta mixes, processed cheeses, salted snack foods, seasoned salt, soy sauce
Low-sodium foods	Fresh fruits and vegetables, fresh meat, fresh poultry, fresh seafood, plain frozen vegetables, fruit juice, herbs/spices, rice/pasta, unsalted cereals, unsalted crackers
Magnesium-rich foods	Apples, bananas, brown rice, dried fruits (especially figs), fish, ginger root, whole grains, grapefruit, green vegetables, lamb, lemons, nuts (especially almonds, brazils, cashews), seafood
Iron-rich foods	Asparagus, dark green vegetables and salad foods, dried fruit, free-range eggs, peppers, lamb's liver, oatmeal, parsley, pulses, seafood, watercress. *Absorption is enhanced if vitamin C is taken at the same time.*
Vitamin K-rich foods	Kelp, all green leafy vegetables, tomatoes, whole grain cereals, liver, cheese, egg yolk, some fruits, and milk

FOOD TYPE	FOOD SOURCES
Vitamin D-rich foods	Cod-liver oil, free-range eggs, mackerel, salmon, sardines, tuna. *Also produced by the action of ultraviolet light on the skin*
Vitamin A-rich foods	Butter, cheese, cod-liver oil, free-range eggs, halibut-liver oil, lamb's liver, oily fish
Vitamin B-rich foods	Apricots, avocado, bananas, brown rice, carrots, chicken, dried fruits, free-range eggs, whole grains, lamb's kidney, melon, nuts, oats, oily fish, potatoes, pumpkin, root and green vegetables, rye flour, salad produce, yogurt
Vitamin C-rich foods	Broccoli, brussels sprouts, cabbage, cauliflower, cherries, grapefruits, kale, kiwi fruits, lemons, mustard and cress, sprouted lentils, parsley, peppers, rosehips, potatoes, tomatoes, watercress. *Oranges are excluded because they can cause allergic reactions and stomach pain in some people.*
Vitamin E-rich foods	Linseeds, sunflower seeds, apples, bananas, broccoli, brown rice, brussels sprouts, carrots, cashew nuts, free-range eggs, whole grains, lamb's liver, nuts, onions, salmon, shrimp, spinach
Foods that acidify urine	Eggs, peanuts, meat, chicken, vitamin C (greater than 5 grams per day), and wheat-containing foods
Foods that alkalinize urine	Dairy products, nuts, vegetables (except corn and lentils), and most fruits
Acid-Alkaline balance	Proteins tend to increase the acidity of the blood, and fruits and vegetables make the blood more alkaline.
Foods containing tyramine	Beer, ale, robust red wines, Chianti, vermouth, homemade breads, cheese, crackers (with cheese), sour cream, bananas, red plums, figs, raisins, avocados, fava beans, Italian broad beans, green bean pods, eggplant, pickled herring, sausages, canned meats, salami, yogurt, soup cubes, commercial gravies, chocolate, and soy sauce

Potassium is an intracellular cation that plays an essential role in maintaining the acid–base and water balance in the body. A proper balance between sodium, calcium, and potassium is necessary for proper cardiac function. Increased levels of potassium result in tall tented T waves. Decreased levels of potassium result in ST depression and U waves.

Calcium is the primary mineral needed for building and maintaining strong bones. Calcium is important to growing children (peak bone-building years are between the teens and early 30s) and women. Calcium helps to prevent osteoporosis, which can occur in women after menopause. Increased levels of calcium result in shortened QT intervals. Decreased levels of calcium result in lengthening of the QT intervals.

Potassium and calcium are directly related to a healthy functioning heart. Increased or decreased levels of potassium or calcium can adversely affect the heart with dangerous arrhythmias.

Sodium is the major extracellular cation and determines the osmolality of the extracellular fluid. Decreased levels of serum sodium concentration are associated with diarrhea, vomiting, syndrome of inappropriate antidiuretic hormone (SIADH), the late stages of congestive heart failure and cirrhosis, acute or chronic renal failure, and diuretic therapy. Increased levels of serum sodium concentration are associated with insensible water loss that is not replaced by drinking (comatose patient with diabetes insipidus).

Iron is important to the human body because it is the main component of hemoglobin. A small but constant intake of iron is necessary to replace erythrocytes that are destroyed in the body. Iron deficiency anemia is the most common form of anemia but loss of blood from bleeding ulcers, hemorrhoids, or injury may also result in a deficiency of iron.

Vitamin K promotes blood clotting by increasing the synthesis of prothrombin by the liver. A deficiency of Vitamin K results in delayed clotting and results in excessive bleeding and bruising under the skin.

Vitamin D is obtained from the direct action of sunlight on the skin that changes certain substances in the body into Vitamin D. Vitamin D is required for the utilization of calcium and phosphorus (essential components for growth and maintenance of healthy bones). Vitamin D deficiencies result in rickets in children and osteomalacia and osteoporosis in adults.

Antidotes for Selected Drugs

DRUG	ANTIDOTE
Acetaminophen	Acetylcysteine
Anticholinesterases (cholinergics)	Atropine, pralidoxime
Antidepressants (MAO inhibitors and tyramine-containing foods may lead to hypertensive crisis including symptoms of chest pain, severe headache, nuchal rigidity, nausea and vomiting, photosensitivity, and enlarged pupils)	Phentolamine
Benzodiazepines	Flumazenil
Cyanide	Amyl nitrite, sodium nitrite, sodium thiosulfate
Digoxin, digitoxin	Digoxin immune fab (Digibind)
Fluorouracil (5FU)	Leucovorin calcium
Heparin	Protamine sulfate
Ifosfamide (Adverse effects cause hemorrhagic cystitis)	Mesna
Iron	Deferoxamine
Lead	Edetate calcium disodium, dimercaprol, succimer
Methotrexate (Adverse effects cause folic acid deficiency)	Leucovorin calcium
Opioid analgesics, heroin	Nalmefene, naloxone
Thrombolytic agents	Aminocaproic acid (Amicar)
Tricyclic antidepressants	Physostigmine
Warfarin (Coumadin)	Phytonadione (vitamin K)

IV Complications

COMPLICATION	SIGNS AND SYMPTOMS
Infiltration	Coolness, edema at site, sluggish flow rate
Phlebitis	Pain or tenderness along the vein with erythema, edema, and warmth
Extravasation	Severe pain during infusion, erythema and edema at the insertion site, and sluggish flow rate
Pyrogenic shock	Sudden increase in temperature, chills, headache, and backache
Circulatory overload	Increased blood pressure, respiratory distress, dilation of neck veins, cough, crackles, and pulmonary edema
Thrombophlebitis	Warm red streak, pain, edema at site, and sluggish flow rate
Air embolism	Decreased blood pressure, weak and rapid pulse, and cyanosis
Speed shock	Headache, irregular pulse, flushed face, syncope, and tightness in the chest

IV Solutions (Hypertonic, Hypotonic, and Isotonic)

ISOTONIC	HYPERTONIC	HYPOTONIC
0.9% normal saline (NS or NaCl) Used to treat hypovolemia Used to correct sodium and chloride deficiencies Used to treat mild metabolic alkalosis **Only** solution used to administer blood products	Dextrose in water (10% and 50%) Used to prevent and treat ketosis Used for hypoglycemic episodes	0.45% normal saline (NS or NaCl) Used to treat mild metabolic alkalosis Replaces sodium, chloride, and free water
Lactated Ringers (LR) Used to treat hypovolemia Used to correct fluid and electrolyte deficiencies Used to treat mild metabolic acidosis	Dextrose 5% in 0.45% normal saline Used to promote renal function and excretion	0.25% normal saline (NS or NaCl) Used to treat hypernatremia
Dextrose 5% in Water (D5W) Used to prevent and treat ketosis Used to prevent dehydration Used to correct hypoglycemia Used to supply water Used to treat high potassium with insulin	Dextrose 5% in normal saline Used to treat fluid volume deficit Used for daily maintenance of body fluids and nutrition	
Dextrose 5% in 0.25% normal saline Used to treat hypernatremia Used for daily maintenance of body fluids (Na and Cl)		

Quick Reference Head-to-Toe Assessment

SYSTEM	ASSESSMENT
Central nervous system (CNS)	• Assess level of consciousness (time, place, person) • Assess vital signs (monitor for signs of increased ICP) • Assess pupils for PEARLA • Assess motor ability (strength and movement) • Assess sensory function (numbness, tingling, or burning) • Discuss history of CNS disease • Discuss CNS medication history • Review CNS diagnostics
Cardiovascular	• Assess pulse for rate, rhythm, and volume • Assess blood pressure (compare extremities) • Auscultate heart sounds • Inspect neck veins for distention • Assess peripheral pulses (compare extremities) • Inspect for peripheral edema • Assess skin color, mucous membranes, and nailbeds • Discuss history of cardiovascular disease • Discuss cardiovascular medication history • Review cardiovascular diagnostics
Respiratory	• Assess skin color and note change in relation to activity • Assess respiratory rate, rhythm, quality, and effort • Observe for tracheal position • Inspect for use of accessory muscles • Describe cough and sputum • Observe for signs of cerebral impairment • Auscultate lung sounds and symmetry • Note change in behavior • Discuss history of respiratory disease • Discuss respiratory medication history • Review respiratory diagnostics

SYSTEM	ASSESSMENT
Gastrointestinal	• Assess abdominal contour and color • Assess for nausea, vomiting, and diarrhea • Auscultate bowel sounds • Palpate abdomen for masses • Discuss bowel patterns (movements and flatus) • Assess appetite and changes in weight • Discuss history of gastrointestinal disease • Discuss gastrointestinal medication history • Review gastrointestinal diagnostics
Urinary	• Assess pattern of voiding (amount, color, clarity, and odor) • Assess for dysuria, urgency, frequency, hesitancy, or hematuria • Palpate bladder for distention • Assess for flank pain • Discuss history of urinary disease • Discuss urinary medication history • Review urinary diagnostics
Integumentary	• Assess skin for general appearance, color, turgor, and integrity • Observe for venous or arterial obstruction • Observe for peripheral edema • Assess temperature of skin • Assess for abnormalities (petechiae, ecchymosis, purpura) • Discuss history of integumentary disease • Discuss integumentary medication history • Review integumentary diagnostics
Musculoskeletal	• Note absence of limbs or digits • Assess range of joint motion • Assess for joint pain or stiffness • Assess for muscle pain, cramps, or spasms • Assess weight bearing and gait pattern • Assess Homans' sign • Discuss history of bone or joint disease • Discuss musculoskeletal medication history • Review musculoskeletal diagnostics

SYSTEM	ASSESSMENT
Psychosocial	• Discuss feelings in regard to health • Assess for anxiety, depression, or mood changes • Discuss adequacy of support system and concerns • Discuss coping strategies (effective and ineffective) • Discuss history of psychosocial disease • Discuss psychosocial medication history • Review psychosocial diagnostics

IICP, increased intracranial pressure; PEARLA, pupils equal and react to light and accommodation.